Small Animal Practice

With the compliments of

KATHARINE HINTON
Publishing Manager

BAILLIERE TINDALL LIMITED

Harcourt Brace Jovanovich, Publishers

24-28 OVAL ROAD, LONDON NW1 7DX, U.K.

TELEPHONE: 071-267 4466 FACSIMILE: 071-482 2293 TELEX: 25775 ACPRES G

The *In Practice* Handbooks Series

Series Editor: Edward Boden

Past and present members of *In Practice* Editorial Board

Professor J. Armour, Chairman 1979–1989,
Dean, Veterinary Faculty, University of Glasgow

P.B. Clarke
Professor L. B. Jeffcott
J. Richardson
S. A. Hall
Professor M. J. Clarkson
Dr W. M. Allen
B. Martin
K. Urquhart
Dr P. G. Darke
S. D. Gunn (Chairman 1990–)
I. Baker
A. Duncan
Professor G. B. Edwards

Titles in print:
Feline Practice
Canine Practice
Equine Practice
Bovine Practice
Sheep and Goat Practice
Swine Practice
Small Animal Practice
Poultry Practice
Equine Practice 2

The *In Practice* Handbooks

Small Animal Practice

Edited by E. Boden
Executive Editor, *In Practice*

Baillière Tindall

LONDON   PHILADELPHIA   TORONTO   SYDNEY   TOKYO

Baillière Tindall   24–28 Oval Road
W. B. Saunders   London NW1 7DX

The Curtis Center
Independence Square West
Philadelphia, PA 19106–3399, USA

55 Horner Avenue
Toronto, Ontario, M8Z 4X6, Canada

Harcourt Brace Jovanovich Group
(Australia) Pty Ltd
30–52 Smidmore Street
Marrickville
NSW 2204, Australia

Harcourt Brace Jovanovich Japan Inc
Ichibancho Central Building
22–1 Ichibancho
Chiyoda-ku, Tokyo 102, Japan

© 1993 Baillière Tindall

Typeset by Photo-graphics, Honiton, Devon
Printed and bound in Hong Kong by Dah Hua Printing Press Co., Ltd.

A catalogue record for this book is available from
the British Library

ISBN 0–7020 1685–3

Contents

Contributors   ix

Foreword   xi

1   **Acute trauma in small animals 1: initial**   1
   assessment and management: J. Foster
   Introduction. Basic requirements. Assessment.
   Case management. Treatment procedures. History
   taking. Specific problems

2   **Acute trauma in small animals 2: thoracic**   23
   injuries: J. E. F. Houlton
   Introduction. Radiography. Thoracocentesis. Types
   of chest injuries. Conclusions

3   **Acute trauma in small animals 3: orthopaedic**   47
   injuries: H. Denny
   Introduction. Head injury. Spinal injury.
   Orthopaedic injuries—examination. Basic
   management of dislocations. First aid procedures
   for temporary immobilization of fractures or
   injured joints. The appropriate method of fracture
   fixation

4   **Acute trauma in small animals 4: abdominal**   65
   injuries: H. Pearson
   Introduction. Types of abdominal injury. Solid
   organ trauma. Hollow organ rupture

5 **Free skin grafting in small animals:** 75
N. McGlennon and R. A. S. White
Introduction. What are the indications for an
FSG? What type of tissue will accept FSGs? How
are FSGs harvested? How are FSGs prepared and
applied? How does an FSG take? What factors
will interfere with the take of FSGs? What
happens to an FSG after it has taken? Conclusion

6 **Fracture fixation in small animal practice:** 91
H. Denny
Introduction. Selection of appropriate method of
fixation. Management of fractures in growing
animals. Fracture treatment in adult animals

7 **External support for small animals:** A. C. Stead 113
Introduction. First aid and postoperative support.
Fracture reduction. Under-cast padding. General
principles of cast application. Casting materials.
Thomas splints. Postoperative care. Cast
complications. Avian fractures

8 **Non-manual restraint of small animals for X-ray:** 131
F. Barr and J. Latham
Introduction. Correct positioning

9 **Chemical restraint for radiography in dogs and** 137
cats: P. M. Taylor
Introduction. Sedatives: use with care. Drug
combinations. Short-acting intravenous
anaesthetics

10 **Diagnostic ultrasound in small animals:** F. Barr 147
Introduction. Equipment. Procedure. Principles of
image interpretation. Applications of diagnostic
ultrasound. General thorax. Conclusion

11 **Blood sampling in the dog and cat:** 169
M. W. Patteson and P. D. Williams
Introduction. Preparation. Cephalic sampling.
Jugular sampling. Alternatives

Contents   vii

12 **Bone marrow aspiration and biopsy in dogs and**   177
    cats: J. Dunn
    Introduction. Indications. Techniques. Aspiration.
    Core biopsy. Complications

13 **Thoracocentesis in the dog and cat:**   189
    H. C. Rutgers
    Introduction. Preparation. Technique. Sample
    handling and clinicopathologic evaluation

14 **A clinical approach to the management of skin**   197
    tumours in the dog and cat: J. M. Dobson and
    N. T. Gorman
    Introduction. Definitions. Clinical approach to
    cutaneous neoplasms. History. Diagnosis. Therapy
    for cutaneous neoplasms. Specific tumour types

15 **Oral tumours in dogs and cats:** J. M. Dobson and   223
    R. A. S. White
    Introduction. Clinical approach. Primary tumour.
    Detection of local and distant metastases.
    Principles of therapy for oral tumours. Specific
    oral tumours. Differential diagnosis of oral
    tumours. Summary

16 **Hormonal alopecia in dogs and cats:** K. P. Baker   245
    Introduction. Hypothyroidism.
    Hyperadrenocorticism. Pituitary dwarfism. Growth
    hormone responsive alopecia. Sertoli cell tumour.
    Male feminizing syndrome. Progesterone-induced
    alopecia. Female hyperoestrogenism (ovarian
    imbalance type 1). Female hypooestrogenism
    (ovarian imbalance type 2). Female hormonal
    alopecia. Diabetes mellitus. Acanthosis nigricans

17 **Diabetes mellitus:** E. Milne   263
    Introduction. Normal endocrine pancreas.
    Aetiology. History. Clinical signs. Differential
    diagnosis. Diagnosis. Treatment. Discharging the
    diabetic. Investigation of instability. Management
    during surgery. Prognosis

18 **Clinical use of neuromuscular blocking agents in**   281
    dogs and cats: G. J. Brouwer
    Introduction. Achieving muscle relaxation.
    Indications. Contraindications. Neuromuscular
    blocking drugs. Clinical features in the use of
    neuromuscular blocking agents. Principal
    considerations in relaxant anaesthetic techniques.
    Technique of relaxant anaesthesia. Summary

19 **Behavioural problems in dogs and cats:**   301
    V. O'Farrell
    Introduction. General causes of behavioural
    problems. Treatment. Specific disorders in dogs
    and cats. Failure of treatment

Index   321

Contributors

K. P. Baker, Faculty of Veterinary Medicine, Veterinary College Ireland, Ballsbridge, Dublin 4, Ireland

F. Barr, University of Bristol Veterinary School, Department of Veterinary Surgery, Langford House, Langford, Bristol BS18 7DU, UK

G. J. Brouwer, Home Office Inspector, E Division, 9th Floor, Tower Block, Home Office, 50 Queen Anne's Gate, London SW1H 9AT, UK

H. Denny, Cedar House, High Street, Wrington, Bristol, Avon BS18 7QD, UK

J. M. Dobson, University of Cambridge, Department of Clinical Veterinary Medicine, Madingley Road, Cambridge CB3 0ES, UK

J. Dunn, Department of Clinical Veterinary Medicine, University of Cambridge, Madingley Road, Cambridge CB3 0ES, UK

J. Foster, Barton Veterinary Hospital, 34 New Dover Road, Canterbury CT1 3DT, UK

N. T. Gorman, University of Glasgow Veterinary School, Department of Veterinary Surgery, Bearsden Road, Bearsden, Glasgow G61 1QH, UK

J. E. F. Houlton, University of Cambridge, Department of Clinical Veterinary Medicine, Madingley Road, Cambridge CB3 0ES, UK

J. Latham, University of Bristol Veterinary School, Department of Veterinary Surgery, Langford House, Langford, Bristol BS18 7DU, UK

N. McGlennon, Ciba-Geigy Agrochemicals, Whittlesford, Cambridge, Cambs CB2 4QT, UK

E. Milne, Royal (Dick) School of Veterinary Studies, Department of Veterinary Medicine, Veterinary Field Station, Easterbush, Roslin, Midlothian EH25 9RG, UK

V. O'Farrell, Royal (Dick) School of Veterinary Studies, Department of Veterinary Clinical Studies, Summerhall, Edinburgh EH9 1QH, UK

M. W. Patteson, University of Bristol Veterinary School, Department of Veterinary Surgery, Langford House, Langford, Bristol BS18 7DU, UK

H. Pearson, University of Bristol Veterinary School, Langford House, Langford, Bristol BS18 7DU, UK

H. C. Rutgers, The Royal Veterinary College, Department of Small Animal Medicine, Hawkshead Lane, North Mymms, Hatfield, Herts AL9 7TA, UK

A. C. Stead, Royal (Dick) School of Veterinary Studies, Department of Veterinary Clinical Studies, Summerhall, Edinburgh EH9 1QH, UK

P. M. Taylor, Animal Health Trust, P.O. Box 5, Newmarket, Suffolk CB8 7DW, UK

R. A. S. White, Division of Surgery, Department of Clinical Veterinary Medicine, University of Cambridge, Madingley Road, Cambridge CB3 0ES, UK

P. D. Williams, 8 Quantock Rise, Kingston St Mary, Taunton, Somerset TA2 8HJ, UK

Foreword

In Practice was started in 1979 as a clinical supplement to *The Veterinary Record*. Its carefully chosen, highly illustrated articles specially commissioned from leaders in their field were aimed specifically at the practitioner. In the form of 'opinionated reviews', they have proved extremely popular with experienced veterinarians and students alike. The editorial board, chaired for the first 10 years by Professor James Armour, was particularly concerned to emphasize differential diagnosis.

In response to consistent demand, articles from *In Practice*, updated and revised by the authors, are now published in convenient handbook form. Each book deals with a particular species or group of related animals.

E. Boden

CHAPTER 1

Acute Trauma in Small Animals 1: Initial Assessment and Management

JOHN FOSTER

INTRODUCTION

Although the word trauma translated from the Greek means "wound", its meaning now has changed to encompass the principle of an injury inflicted by a variable degree of force suddenly, by physical or chemical action. In small animal medicine acute trauma implies a point of crisis common to many emergencies met in everyday practice. Indeed, approximately one in eight admissions for in-patient care is a critically traumatized or injured dog or cat patient.

Of these admissions approximately two-thirds will have been involved in road traffic accidents. The pet dog is normally a more closely monitored animal than the pet cat. Whereas the cause and origin of the trauma for the critically injured cat is in the main unknown, more than half the dogs will have been seen to have been involved in a collision with a motor vehicle. Thus the time, nature, severity and site of injury may well be provided in some detail, all of which helps greatly with the assessment, the prognosis and the therapy.

Natural antagonism between members of the same species accounts for the next most common source of acute trauma and then, less frequently, between them, the humans and other domestic species.

In terms of cause and incidence the differing lifestyles of cats and dogs do obviously play a part in the injuries incurred. The cat, being a climber, not infrequently falls off a roof or out of a window, whereas the dog, less cautious on the ground, will meet sharp objects. Crush injuries and burns and scalds are seen least frequently, but nevertheless form a significant percentage of admissions under the "critically injured" classification.

BASIC REQUIREMENTS

The nature of the critically injured patient does not permit, in general, the luxury of sufficient time to locate and consider in depth the application of resuscitative techniques, the administration of life saving drugs or the organization of supportive therapy equipment.

Therefore the practice must make a conscious decision to equip a room or part of a room, preferably away from the general public areas, with:

(1)   A versatile resuscitative and anaesthetic apparatus capable of intermittent positive pressure ventilation
(2)   An easily accessible and full range of cuffed and small size uncuffed endotracheal tubes
(3)   Items for intravenous short- and long-stay catheterization (Figs 1.1 and 1.2)
(4)   Various intravenous fluids, including specific replacement solutions (dextrose 5%, Hartmann's or Ringer's-lactate), plasma volume expanders (dextrans and gelatin/urea compounds), whole blood or plasma, and fluids for specific therapy (mannitol, sodium bicarbonate solution), infusions scales and drip stands
(5)   Urinary catheters and collection bags, a suction apparatus, basic sterile surgical instrument packs, blankets or insulated bedding, hot water bottles and/or a heating pad.

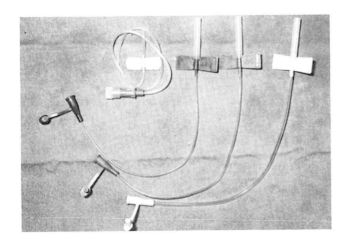

Fig. 1.1
Cannulae for short-term intravenous access. From left to right: Abbott Butterfly—25 (0.5 mm), Portex Minivens 23 gauge (blue), 21 gauge (green), 19 gauge (white).

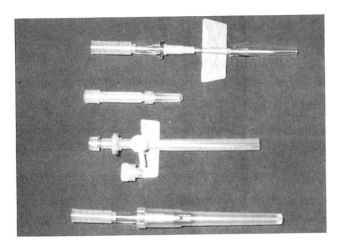

Fig. 1.2
Cannulae for long-term intravenous access; over-the-needle type. From top to bottom: Angio Set Shorty 20 gauge × 1 inch (Deseret), PRN Adaptor (Deseret), Venflon i/v cannula LL-26 (Venflon), Angio catheter 16 gauge × 2 inch (Deseret).

DRUGS

Located in this emergency facility or nearby in a position known to all staff should be a drug box ("Mayday" box) (Fig. 1.3 and Table 1.1) containing basic essentials for therapeutic resuscitation.

A contents list and a dosage chart need to be attached to it so that its stock content can always be maintained and dosages of infrequently used drugs will not have to be researched. (Tables 1.2 and 1.3)

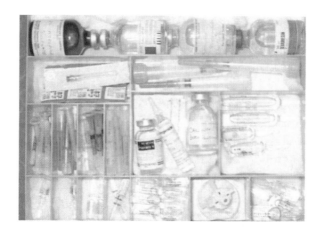

Fig. 1.3
"Mayday" box containing essentials for therapeutic resuscitation. Adapted from fishing tackle box.

Table 1.1 "Mayday" box: first aid instructions to nurses.

Cardiac arrest is a three minute emergency

Instructions

(1) Establish airway—absolute priority
(2) Ventilate lungs—oxygen if possible, air if not and mouth to tube if needs be
(3) External heart massage—not too rapid, allow time for ventricular filling

Lay staff do not proceed beyond this point

(4) Internal heart massage—wet hair with 1% Savlon solution, *do not* stop to clip up or scrub up. Incise fifth intercostal space either side, preferably left
(5) Inject calcium borogluconate or calcium chloride into ventricle
(6) Inject diluted adrenalin solution intravenously (not peripheral vein)
(7) Continue massage and ventilation

Establish venepuncture(s) in largest vein(s) available, ie, jugular

(8) Correct acidosis with sodium bicarbonate solution, two doses during crisis then half doses at 10 min intervals

Some basic rules have to be remembered. The administration of sedatives and analgesics in the acute trauma case is hazardous unless the cause has been established and found to be compatible with this therapy. Diazepam intravenously as a mild ataractic in dogs and cats will not cause as profound

Table 1.2 "Mayday box": typical contents.

Contents	Type	Size		Quantity
Syringes	Disposable	Plastic	2 ml	5
			5 ml	2
			10 ml	2
Needles	Disposable		21 gauge $\times \frac{5}{8}$ inch	10
			21 gauge $\times 1\frac{1}{2}$ inch	5
			18 gauge $\times 1\frac{1}{2}$ inch	10
Miniven (Portex)	Luer	White	19 gauge	2
		Green	21 gauge	2
		Blue	23 gauge	2
Intravenous catheters	Angio Set Shorty (Deseret)		20 gauge $\times$ 1 inch	2
			22 gauge $\times \frac{3}{4}$ inch	2
PRN adaptors	(Deseret)			2
Three-way tap (Braun)	Disposable			1

Drugs		Concentration	Size	Quantity
Adrenaline tartrate		1:1000	1 ml	5
Atropine sulphate		0.5 mg/ml	30 ml	1
Bemegride (Megimide; Nicholas)		5 mg/ml	10 ml	2
Calcium borogluconate		10%	50 ml	1
Calcium chloride		10%	50 ml	1
Dexamethasone (Dexadreson; Intervet)		2 mg/ml	50 ml	1
Doxapram hydrochloride (Dopram-V; A. H. Robins)		20 mg/ml	20 ml	1
Lignocaine HCl (no adrenaline)		2%	50 ml	1
Methylprednisolone sodium succinate (Solu-Medrone V; Upjohn)		500 mg	8 ml	2
Naloxone hydrocholoride (Narcan; Winthrop)		0.4 mg/ml	1 ml	2
Nikethamide (Evans Medical)		25%	2 ml	5
Potassium chloride		20%	5 ml	5
Procaine hydrochloride (no adrenaline)		2%	50 ml	1
Sodium bicarbonate		4.2%	50 ml	1
Water for injection			100 ml	1

Table 1.3 "Mayday" box: drug dosages.

Drug	Dose	Route
Acepromazine	0.55 mg/kg	i/m, i/v, s/c
Adrenaline tartrate 1:1000	Dilute 1 ml in 9 ml water then 1–4 ml	i/v, i/cardiac
Atropine sulphate	0.05 mg/kg	i/m, i/v, s/c
Bemegride	up to 10 ml every 3–4 minutes	i/v
Buprenorphine hydrochloride	0.006–0.02 mg/kg	i/m, i/v
Calcium borogluconate 10%	5–10 ml	i/cardiac
Calcium chloride 10%	1 ml/10kg	i/cardiac
Choramphenicol	20–50 mgkg	i/v
Crystalline sodium penicillin	1,000,000–1,5000,000 iu/ml i/v solution	i/v
Dexamethasone	4–8 mg/kg	i/v
Doxapram hydrochloride		
Anaesthetic reversal	1–10 mg/kg every 15–20 minutes	i/v
Neonate resuscitation	1–5 mg	sublingual s/c i/v
Digoxin	0.02 mg/kg	slow i/v
Furosemide	5–20 mg/kg	i/v
Gallamine triethiodide	1–2 mg/kg	i/v
Heparin	2 mg/kg	i/v
Isoprotarenol hydrochloride	0.005–0.015 mg/kg, 0.02 mg in 100 ml dilution	i/v
Lignocaine hydrochloride (no adrenaline)	50–100 mg	i/cardiac
Methylprednisolone sodium succinate	20–40 mg/kg	i/v, i/m
Morphine hydrochloride	0.02–0.8 mg/kg	i/v, s/c, i/m
Naloxone hydrochloride	To effect—short acting	i/v, s/c, i/m
Nikethamide	To effect—with caution	i/v
Pentazocine lactate	1–3.5 mg/kg	i/v, i/m, s/c
Pethidine hydrochloride	1–10 mg/kg	i/v, i/m, s/c
Phenergan	20 mg/kg	i/v, i/m
Potassium chloride 4%	1–3 ml	i/v, dilute
Sodium bicarbonate	1–3 mEq/kg (500 ml of 5% = 300 mEq), ie, 50 ml/10kg	i/v

i/v intravenous, i/m intramuscular, i/cardiac intraventricular, s/c subcutaneous

a depression of blood pressure as phenothiazine derivatives, but in all cases treatment or prevention of shock must be considered hand in hand. Narcotics or opiates are contraindicated in head injuries but if an analgesic is required pentazocine may be given to the dog for other, mainly orthopaedic injuries.

Should the packed cell volume fall below 0.25 litres/litre whole blood is the best replacement fluid. Fluid and electrolytes may be administered to the hypovolaemic patient rapidly at the rate of 3 ml/kg/min for the initial 10 min. As much as 30–90 ml/kg bodyweight may be administered to save life, assuming cardiopulmonary function remains unimpaired.

Corticoids work best at a normal blood pH value. Large doses of corticoids with low pHs (dexamethasone, pH 4.1) may therefore delay reaction time, so it is best to administer this drug first well diluted and secondly with bicarbonate solution. Mannitol is a potent non-renal osmotic diuretic useful especially in cranial injuries producing neural oedema, but it should not be used until hypovolaemia is corrected. A "rebound" effect on blood pressure a few hours later should be anticipated.

The success of the support for the circulation can be carried out by a series of laboratory examinations, including the measurements of central venous pressure, but for most practices the absolute minimum of monitoring should be directed towards packed cell volume and urinary output volume.

STAFF

Critical care from the point of initial emergency treatment through continuous monitoring to stabilization of the animal is a commitment which will involve a great deal of time and effort from both the nursing and, to a lesser extent, veterinary staff. No case will illustrate better the nature of team work in veterinary medicine. Therefore instruction of staff is paramount and each will know his or her place in the group to work around or on a patient. In the absence of professional staff, the nurse must be made aware of what he or she may or may not do.

All must appreciate the rudiments of the assessment of injury, not only to forward the information if needs be, but to know when and what to apply from basic first aid to more sophisticated techniques under direction or supervision.

ASSESSMENT

More than 65% of cases requiring critical care are likely to be
road traffic accidents and therefore trauma may be considerable. Of these many will show injury to more than one part
of the body.

On presentation the historical details are of minimal
importance. The few important facts can be acquired while
the animal is subjected to a prescribed systematic primary
assessment. Only the "when" of the accident transcends
other thoughts about the history. From this small piece of
information flows the severity and prognosis for the level of
consciousness, the degree of shock or the capacity of the
cardiopulmonary system to cope.

Ideally, the animal should not be stressed further, and this
applies especially to cats whose wish in shock is to seek
seclusion.

Assuming that by this rapid evaluation the animal's survival
is not compromised, ie, there is no immediate or severe
respiratory or cardiovascular embarrassment, then a general
examination will reveal: any obvious abnormalities in body
conformation; evidence of external haemorrhage; mucous
membrane and skin colour; the quality and nature of pulse
and respiration; the body core temperature and that of the
extremities; the state of consciousness and the degree of pain
and/or disability.

Now, only if the animal is not acutely critical, the secondary
more detailed assessment can begin. Each examiner should
adopt a set routine for close inspection. For example, start at
the head and check all orifices, the mouth, mucous membranes,
tongue, palate, maxilla and mandible, the position of the eyes
and the sclerae, anterior ocular structures, pupillary size and
reactivity, optic fissure and position of lids and their reflexes.
Next, the ears and superficial ear canals, the head carriage
and degrees of reactivity to sight and sound can be assessed
quickly and easily.

The examination then moves backwards via the neck to the
thorax and abdomen, both superficially and by deep structure
evaluation. An intact bladder, which even in road traffic
accidents can contain an appreciable amount of urine, is a

useful finding, as are those of normal hindlimb reflexes and a good pulse.

The extremities are left until last, but even then in the presence of pain there is little point in subjecting an animal in shock to further abuse to make a palpated diagnosis of a fractured limb bone.

CASE MANAGEMENT

In an ideal veterinary world the in-depth assessment and management of the trauma case would be achieved using data produced from the estimation of central venous pressure, electrocardiography, full haematology and blood biochemistry, urinalysis, cerebrospinal fluid analysis, blood gas analysis and whole body radiography.

But 99% of the cases presented to 99% of the practices in this country now cannot be subjected to this extreme form of monitoring. Much is made of these examinations in texts dealing with critical patient care and thus it may serve to detract from the clinical assessment made by practice members. It is a cardinal sin to ignore obvious vital signs as a result of a premature resort to clinical pathology and the sacrifice of essential time should be devoted to basic life-saving efforts.

Often the trauma case is first seen for one reason or another by a member of the nursing staff. Their protocol should involve knowledge to cope with the following evaluation procedure in order of priority:

(1)   Assess airway sufficiency
(2)   Stem substantial external bleeding
(3)   Assess cardiopulmonary status
(4)   Dress or cover major external wounds
(5)   Assess state of the central nervous system
(6)   Assess bone and joint status
(7)   Make an overall assessment of the animal's wellbeing.

However, this examination must not totally ignore the needs of the owner. Most will be in an emotional state, some even in shock themselves. Therefore most owners will welcome the sight of calm and competent inspection and be soothed by it. Their presence may well be necessary anyway to assist in holding the animal. However, at the first opportunity the owner and patient are best separated, especially if rapid action and therapy is to be undertaken and injuries are to be exposed.

FIRST AID

The nurse should be capable of performing a wide range of tasks under this heading until the veterinary surgeon takes over. In the first instance he or she may have to give directions about transport of the animal from where the trauma took place to the surgery or hospital. Again competent, calm and authoritative advice on how to lift the animal, how to transfer it on to a makeshift stretcher, via box or basket, and by wheeled transport must be given. Owners are often keen to feed trauma cases, so an instruction not to offer food or fluids should be part of the telephone message.

The nurse must warn the veterinary surgeon in charge that an emergency case is on its way and prepare for the tasks of accepting the case, evaluating the position, administering first aid and transferring information to the veterinary surgeon. None of this is achieved without the practice adopting a training programme for all staff.

TREATMENT PROCEDURES

Just as the nursing staff must have an idea of the way to proceed and the limit of what they are permitted to do, so must there be a protocol by which the professional continues with the case. This is indicated in Table 1.4.

HISTORY TAKING

Although some of the information on the animal's history will have been obtained already by now, it may be useful to categorise the questions to obtain essential facts which will

Table 1.4 Procedures which the veterinary surgeon should follow when dealing with the acute trauma case.

---

(1) Ensure adequate airway passage patency and that there is sufficient ventilation and oxygenation

(2) Control only severe external bleeding

(3) Establish one or more intravenous cannulae or a combination of short- (hours) and long-stay (days) intravenous access

(4) Establish an intravenous infusion, initially lactated-Ringer's (or Hartmann's) solution perhaps with the addition of bicarbonate, at the dose rate of 40–90 ml/kg bodyweight

(5) Administer intravenous prednisolone sodium succinate (rapid and short acting) and then subsequently dexamethasone (delayed and long acting)

(6) Administer antibiotics intravenously

(7) Take a blood sample for packed cell volume, total blood proteins, blood urea nitrogen and, if possible, electrolyte analysis

(8) Catheterize the urinary bladder and empty it, perform urinalysis and monitor urine production thereafter as a mark of essential cardiovascular and renal function return (normal dog urinary output: 10–20 ml/kg/day)

(9) If capillary refill time is more than two seconds but estimated hypovolaemia has been substantially corrected, peripheral resistance may need to be relieved by using a beta-adrenergic blocker such as chlorpromazine

(10) Assuming signs of restlessness and hyperventilation are pain related and not caused by hypoxia, administer pentazocine or pethidine

(11) Return to patient monitoring of packed cell volume, total blood proteins, urine output, body temperature, pulse and respiration rate and quality, capillary refill time and membrane colour, and, perhaps, ECG. (Note that if the body temperature falls below 34°C the mechanism associated with hypothermia cannot operate, so external heat is required which includes a warmed intravenous infusion)

(12) A further rapid but more detailed general physical examination with the order of priority of: respiratory system, cardiovascular system, abdomen, soft tissues including central and peripheral nervous systems, fractures and dislocations.
At this stage the owner needs to be informed again of progress. Now a more relevant prognosis can be given and at the same time the remainder of the history of the animal gleaned.

---

influence mainly the prognosis and to some extent continued treatment.

Of immediate interest are:

(1) What happened? Did you see the injury take place? Where did it happen?

(2) How long ago did the trauma occur?

(3) Was the animal fully conscious after the trauma, and has it remained so since?

(4) Has the animal's condition improved, stayed the same or become worse since the trauma?

(5) Did the animal walk after the trauma and how well did it do so?

(6) Did you see any haemorrhage and if so from where?

(7) What have you done in terms of first aid?

and then later:

(8) Are there any other medical or surgical problems and is the animal receiving medication now?

(9) When was the animal last fed and when did it pass urine or faeces?

(10) What is the animal's age and has it been neutered?

The list may seem laborious but the information flows readily and usually involves short answers. One of the most relevant questions relates to age. The more susceptible age groups to shock and control nervous system trauma will be the young and then perhaps the old.

SPECIFIC PROBLEMS

SHOCK

Without doubt the most common pathophysiological occurrence to be dealt with is shock. Shock is a syndrome seen when the cardiovascular system is unable to maintain blood pressure and flow above minimal physiological tissue requirements. In other words there is an acute decline in tissue blood supply.

Of the three categories of shock, cardiogenic, hypovolaemic and vasculogenic, the most commonly met in veterinary practice is hypovolaemic. Vascular constriction in mesenteric, hepatic, cutaneous, muscular and renal blood vessels and blood redistribution towards adrenal, myocardial, brain and hepatic arterial vessels under the influence of sympathoadrenal stimulation attempt to conserve pressure and flow to essential "primary" tissues. However, in time anoxia and hypoxia in vasoconstricted organs produce irreversible cellular decline, principally in the kidney, which results in irreversible shock. It is this phenomenon to which therapy must be addressed vigorously.

As a general rule, and accepting that severe external haemorrhage will obviously produce intense hypovolaemia, traumatized patients are also always hypovolaemic. Trauma to the thorax, abdomen and pelvis causes haemorrhage and sequestration of fluids in those areas. Contributing and influencing factors such as pain, excitement, airway obstruction, pneumothorax and pericardial tamponade must be taken into account.

Signs

The signs of shock encountered in a traumatized animal are listed in Table 1.5.

Table 1.5 Signs of shock.

Tachycardia: dogs more than 150 beats/minute and cats more than 180 beats/minute
Pale and cold mucous membranes
Slowed peripheral capillary refill time
Weak and "thready" main arterial pulses (reduced systolic blood pressure)
Non-palpable peripheral arterial pulses
Cold extremities and collapsed superficial veins
Dry and starched tongue
Oliguria and even anuria
Subnormal temperature and absence of shivering
Increased respiratory rate with altered depth
Altered consciousness and muscle weakness

Treatment

First institute immediate therapy. Adequate volume replacement is essential, ideally on an "in-kind" principle. Failing that any crystalloid solution through adequate sized needles, preferably intravenous-only cannulae, will be adequate in the short term. Mild haemodilution may be helpful in shock. Once the adequacy of the airway has been established or oxygen administered, more specific intravenous replacement and drug therapy can be instituted. The colloid/crystalloid combination will be adequate in most cases even where whole blood loss has occurred. The advantage of the use of corticosteroid in hypovolaemia is still equivocal, but nonetheless has not been demonstrated to be harmful.

Avoid any excessive movement. The shock case has much diminished reflex compensatory mechanisms. In particular, the myocardium's failure to maintain output in the face of insult from depressant drugs, which include anaesthetics, must be remembered.

Delay the use of analgesics and, especially, sedatives. Their use before correction of hypovolaemia may precipitate a sudden decrease in peripheral resistance and a catastrophic fall in blood pressure.

The shock case will not tolerate and probably does not even need deep planes of anaesthesia. No surgical interference is indicated before the airway is established, severe external haemorrhage is controlled and volume replacement commenced.

Do not skimp on therapy or neglect the need to monitor the case continuously until stabilization. Nursing care comes into a prime position in shock.

BRAIN, SPINAL CORD AND PERIPHERAL
NERVOUS SYSTEM DAMAGE (Figs. 1.4 and 1.5,
Table 1.6)

Brain damage

In acute trauma cases almost twice as many cats as dogs suffer from head injuries and, comparatively, the dog is more

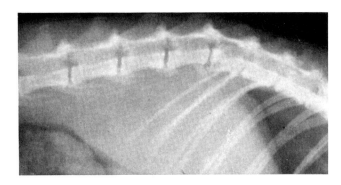

Fig. 1.4
Acute spinal cord
trauma. Fracture of
L1 vertebra. Cat
following a road
traffic accident.

resistant than the cat to intracranial damage. Unconsciousness, semi-consciousness, mild concussive signs and upper motor neuron damage are still frequently seen.

As with shock the immediacy of response to therapy will dictate survival and retention of neurological function to a large degree.

The basic nursing instructions are thus:

(1) Move the animal on a firm flat carrier if possible. Instruct owner as necessary
(2) Ensure a patent airway free from blood, mucus and vomitus
(3) Perform tracheal intubation/cannulation, tracheotomy and oxygenation

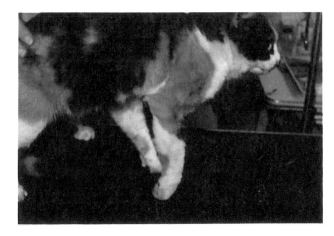

Fig. 1.5
Typical posture of a
cat with radial nerve
paralysis.

Table 1.6 Nervous system signs and spinal innervations.

Clinical signs	Area of damage
Horner's syndrome	Cervical (C7–T1)
Forelimb signs	C6–T1
Diaphragm paralysis	C5, 6, 7
Panniculus reflex	T1–L3
Segmental intercostal paralysis	Thoracic
Hindlimb signs	L3–S2
Atonic bladder	S1–3

(4)   Administer fluid therapy but with caution since hypotension, hypoventilation and overhydration may aggravate cerebral oedema
(5)   Watch central nervous system vital signs, including state of consciousness, pupil sizes and responses, posture and motor functions, vision, character of respiration and presence of convulsions. Determine therapy including the administration of mannitol, corticoids, anticonvulsants (clonazepam and diazepam) and, only if definitely indicated, other sedatives and narcotics.

Spinal cord and peripheral nervous system

A basic working knowledge of neuroanatomy is easily acquired and essential in order to offer a prognosis over the post trauma critical period of 48 h. The principal areas for concern relate to the cervical and lumbar enlargements and the phrenic nucleus where trauma gives rise to lower motor neurone signs of defects in sensation, muscle paralysis with neurogenic atrophy, and diminished spinal reflexes. The peripheral nervous system examination will take place as part of the spinal neurological examination. Charts can be useful if readily available in the emergency room and these are illustrated in Figs 1.6 and 1.7.

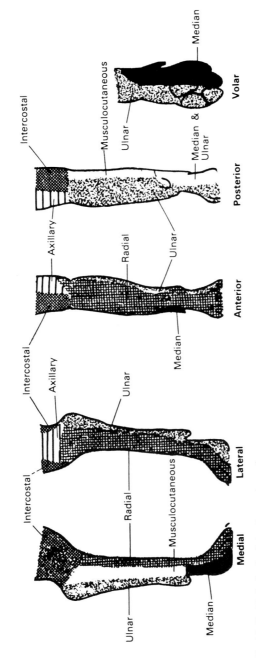

Fig. 1.6 Chart indicating forelimb cutaneous innervations.

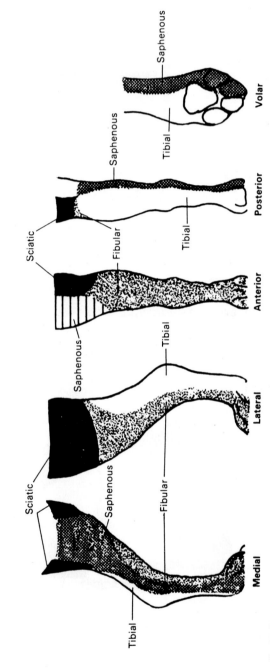

Fig. 1.7 Chart indicating hindlimb cutaneous innervations.

Table 1.7 Common signs of ocular trauma.

Hyphema, plasmoid aqueous (fibrin) and iridodialysis
Chemosis and conjunctival haemorrhage
Episcleral haemorrhage
Epistaxis and adnexal tears, contusions and orbital fractures
Proptosis of the globe, strabismus or paralysis of bulbar muscles
Anisocoria, miosis, mydriasis or unresponsive pupillary light reflex
Bulbar or orbital pain
Corneal tears, penetrations and oedema and iris prolapse
Lens subluxations or luxations
Retinal haemorrhages and retinal detachments
Blindness and/or visual field deficits

OCULAR EMERGENCIES (Table 1.7)

Two facts have to be remembered in trauma to the bulb or
adnexae. First, external trauma may cause severe intraocular
injuries even if the globe is not penetrated. Secondly, post
traumatic uveitis, occurring not infrequently but often not
diagnosed as such, must be controlled (Fig. 1.8).

There is no overall rule to treatment since trauma involving
the globe is likely to give rise to a combination of some of
the above. Certainly proptosis of the bulb is common in the

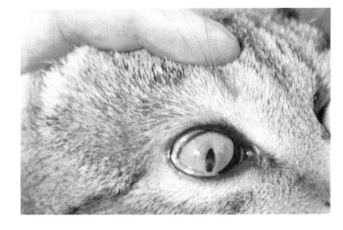

Fig. 1.8
Uveal damage in cat
showing hyphema,
fibrinous exudate,
uveitis and iris
swelling.

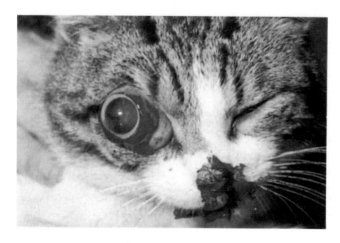

Fig. 1.9
Acute head trauma
with bulbar proptosis,
maxillary fracture with
epistaxis in a cat.

cat and requires immediate medical and surgical care to give any chance of saving the eye (Fig. 1.9).

The medical approach to the above may involve the use of systemic and local corticoids, antibiotics, atropine 1% ointment or drops, and emollients or tear replacement preparations to prevent corneal desiccation.

WOUNDS (Fig. 1.10)

Skin wounds may be minor and superficial or major and deep, few or multiple. Their management, while never, in the absence of severe external haemorrhage, classed as an

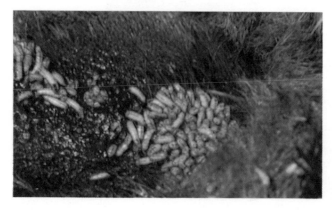

Fig. 1.10
Severe trauma due to
fly strike on lumbar
skin of a Pembroke
corgi bitch.

emergency in nature, involves a proper approach, evaluation and treatment regimen.

The preparation and cleansing of wounds follows a pattern according to the tried and trusted rules of the individual practice. Early wound management is designed to remove contamination, limit infection and scarring and promote early use.

In the author's experience, neglected therapeutic aids such as Vaseline tulle, simply made from gauze swabs heated in petroleum jelly, and PVC drainage tubes enhance results.

BURNS AND SCALDS

Burns used to be classified as first to sixth degree, but these terms may well be now redundant in favour of the simpler terminology of superficial or deep, localized or extensive.

Burns may arise as a result of friction, pure contact heat or cold (frostbite), electrical, chemical, radiation including sunburn, and other causes. All require rapid therapy to limit damage. If more than 15% of the body surface is involved then fluids and electrolytes will be required. Potassium loss in exudation is potentially severe so oral supplementation in the form of potassium gluconate or chloride as well as intravenous physiological saline solution is indicated.

FURTHER READING

Archibald, J., Holt, J. C. & Sokolovsky, V. (1981) *The Management of Trauma in Dogs and Cats*. American Veterinary Publications.

Chandler, E. A., Sutton, J. B. & Thompson, D. J. (1984) *Canine Medicine and Therapeutics*, 2nd edn. Cheltenham, BSAVA Publications.

Kirk, R. W. & Bistner, S. I. (1981) *Handbook of Veterinary Procedures and Emergency Treatment*. Philadelphia, W. B. Saunders & Co.

McDonnell, W. (1974) *Journal of Small Animal Practice* **15**, 293.

Rodkey, W. G. (1980) *Veterinary Clinics of North America* **10**, 56–58.

CHAPTER 2

Acute Trauma in Small Animals 2: Thoracic Injuries

JOHN HOULTON

INTRODUCTION

Unlike many traumatic conditions, chest injuries affect processes which are fundamental to survival. If life is to be maintained, speed, as well as accuracy, is essential in recognizing the nature and extent of the injury. Fortunately, despite the often dramatic nature of the wounds, successful treatment is generally relatively simple.

Trauma has a total disregard for artificially created systems and thoracic injuries cannot be treated in isolation without paying due regard to the remainder of the damage. Nevertheless measures to alleviate respiratory distress should take precedence over everything apart from controlling overt haemorrhage.

In general, surgical management should only be considered after conservative procedures such as thoracocentesis or chest tube drainage have failed to restore adequate alveolar ventilation and perfusion. However, continued leakage of air or blood, in spite of repeated or continuous drainage, necessitates a more aggressive approach. Occasionally, immediate surgery is indicated if the patient is to survive.

RADIOGRAPHY

Thoracic radiographs are important in assessing the nature and extent of the injury. Immediate assessment will demonstrate a pneumothorax or haemothorax but it may be several hours before any pulmonary involvement becomes evident. These pulmonary changes may become more obvious over the subsequent 24–48 h and it is advisable to radiograph the chest daily, or twice daily, if the patient is deteriorating. It is important to keep the exposures constant throughout this serial evaluation in order that any changes in density can be easily interpreted.

Great care must be taken when restraining and positioning any dyspnoeic animal for radiography. Forcible handling must be avoided and the animal should not be rolled on to its back, particularly when the existence of free pleural fluid is suspected. Initially a recumbent lateral projection is taken. The forelegs should be pulled well forwards to reduce superimposition of the upper limb musculature on the cranial thoracic structures and a foam wedge may be used to elevate the sternum so that a true lateral projection is obtained (in this view the costochondral junctions of the two sides of the chest should overlie each other).

An additional dorsoventral projection is generally indicated but positioning is a little more difficult, particularly when there are concomitant upper forelimb fractures. It is important that the chest is not rotated in this view and the sternum and vertebral column should be superimposed on the finished radiograph. Exposure times should be kept as short as possible to reduce respiratory blur and, in general, radiographs should be taken at the peak of inspiration to provide the greatest contrast between the air filled lungs and the other thoracic structures.

THORACOCENTESIS (Figs 2.1 and 2.2)

Thoracocentesis is frequently employed to confirm the existence of intrapleural fluid or air. The chest may be tapped with a catheter attached to a three-way tap and syringe, with

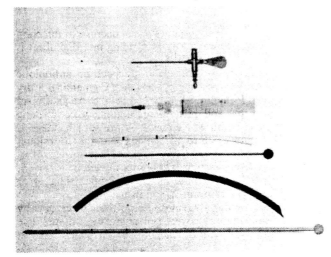

Fig. 2.1
Assorted equipment
for thoracocentesis.

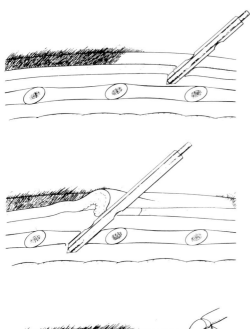

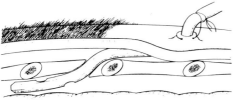

Fig. 2.2
Thoracocentesis using a trochar and
plastic cannula. The subcutaneous
"tunnel" should be 3–5 cm to ensure
an airtight seal.

a trochar and cannula or by the placement of rubber or plastic tubing. The former two are suitable for simple diagnostic drainage but where repeated withdrawal of air or fluid is contemplated a drainage tube is safer.

The site for thoracocentesis is determined by whether air or fluid is to be removed. A pneumothorax is usually drained through the seventh or eighth intercostal space at the mid thoracic level. When fluid is to be drained the ventral third of the same interspace is used.

A chest drain can be inserted under local analgesia by infiltration of the skin, subcutaneous tissues and intercostal muscles. Following routine aseptic preparation a small nick is made in the skin with a scalpel and the drain is tunnelled subcutaneously for 3–5 cm before penetrating the intercostal muscles cranial to the relevant rib. The tube is anchored to the skin with a purse-string suture making sure that sufficient length remains in the chest such that it will not become dislodged during aspiration.

An underwater seal and electrically powered vacuum pump is the ideal way to continuously drain the chest (Fig. 2.3). An added advantage of the underwater seal is that when the pump is disconnected it is possible to assess the intrapleural pressure by measuring the length of the column of water in the tube. Moreover, it is possible to assess the amount of free

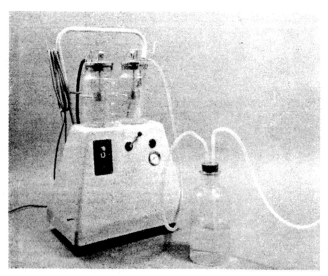

Fig. 2.3
Equipment to enable continuous drainage of the chest. The free end of the drainage tube is attached to a water seal which in turn is attached to an electrically powered vacuum pump. Note the pleural fluid in the drainage tube.

Table 2.1 Different types of thoracic injury following acute trauma.

Disruption of the thoracic wall
Rupture of the diaphragm
Damage to the lung parenchyma
Disruption of the airways
Damage to the heart and vessels
Damage to the oesophagus

air or fluid by measuring the distance that the meniscus travels with each respiration. An unduly large "swing" means further drainage is necessary.

TYPES OF CHEST INJURIES

Damage to the thorax caused by trauma can be divided into six categories (see Table 2.1).

DISRUPTION OF THE THORACIC WALL

Penetrating wounds (Table 2.2)

The most obvious thoracic injury is a penetrating wound of the thoracic wall. Such wounds may be caused by sharp static objects such as stakes or branches or they may be the result

Table 2.2 Signs of penetrating wounds.

Visible wound(s) with possible subcutaneous emphysema
Tachypnoea and dyspnoea
An open pneumothorax with paradoxical breathing

of a dog fight where teeth penetrate the skin and strip away large areas of intercostal tissue (Fig. 2.4).

Subcutaneous emphysema may develop as a result of air entering the wound and collecting under the skin. This emphysema may reach quite dramatic proportions but is rarely dangerous.

Treatment

Initially plug the hole(s) as a first aid measure with a saline moistened pad, or pressure bandage, to alleviate the paradoxical breathing. Then, if necessary, re-expand the lung by simple aspiration.

Once the animal is stable, induce general anaesthesia, institute positive pressure ventilation and assess the full extent of the injuries to the skin, ribs and muscles. Radiography may be helpful in defining the extent of the underlying damage.

All devitalized tissue must be removed before routine surgical closure of the chest wall is effected. It must be appreciated that the size of the skin wound bears no relationship to the extent of the underlying pathology. Where large amounts of damaged intercostal tissue have to be

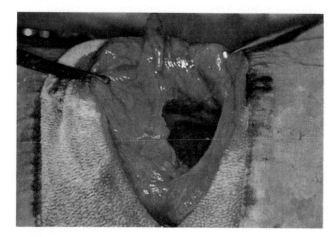

Fig. 2.4
Extensive laceration of the intercostal tissues of a Jack Russell terrier attacked by a larger dog.

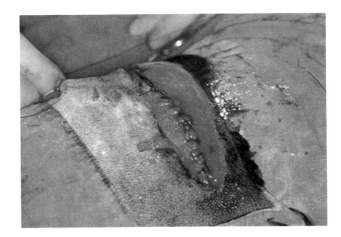

Fig. 2.5
Closure of the chest
wall following a
penetrating wound.
After debridement,
the ribs are coapted
with stainless steel
wire and the
overlying tissues
closed with a
continuous suture.

removed the defect should be made good by coapting adjacent
ribs using wire structures (Fig. 2.5).

Extensive damage to the lung parenchyma will necessitate
a lobectomy or resection of the damaged portion. Subcutaneous
emphysema may take days or weeks to subside but most
cases will resolve with limited exercise.

Flail chest (Table 2.3)

Proximal and distal fractures of two or more adjacent ribs
may result in a section of the chest wall that is free to move
independently of the remainder of the thoracic cage, ie, the
flail segment will collapse inwards on inspiration. Dyspnoea
is often severe owing to the cumulative effect of the paradoxical
breathing and the contusion of the underlying lung tissue.
The greater the inspiratory effort the animal makes the more

Table 2.3 Signs of flail chest.

Dyspnoea
Paradoxical movement of the flail segment
± Other concomitant wounds

Radiography is essential to identify the full extent of the rib fractures
and to assess the damage to the pulmonary parenchyma

damage the flail segment does to the underlying lung parenchyma.

Treatment

First the flail segment should be stabilized to prevent further damage. As a first aid measure the flail segment can be pulled out and held by attaching towel clips to the rib(s).

The affected ribs should then be secured to an external support comprising a frame made of padded aluminium rods contoured to the thoracic wall (Fig. 2.6). The ribs are secured by passing one or more sutures of monofilament nylon or stainless steel wire around each rib and anchoring them to the frame. Care should be taken to avoid the intercostal vessels and nerves which are immediately caudal to the rib.

Alternatively, the flail segment can be immobilized by internal fixation of the rib fractures utilising monofilament stainless steel wire sutures or Kirschner wires. This requires general anaesthesia and intermittent positive pressure ventilation of the patient but may be the treatment of choice if other chest wall defects require simultaneous repair.

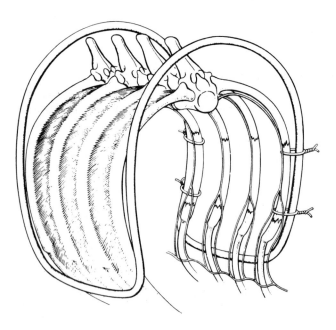

Fig. 2.6
Treating a case of flail chest. The flail segment can be anchored to a padded frame made of aluminium rods. This prevents paradoxical movement of the flail segment.

Non-penetrating wounds

The majority of chest injuries are closed and cause respiratory distress either by introducing foreign matter into the pleural cavity in the form of air, fluid or viscera, or by sequestrating variable amounts of lung tissue by pulmonary oedema or by intrapulmonary haemorrhage.

Rib fractures are a common sequel to blunt thoracic trauma and unless they are associated with other injuries they are often of little clinical significance.

Pain resulting from injury of the chest wall may prevent deep breathing and discourage the animal from coughing. This allows the build up of obstructive secretions within the bronchial tree and may result in respiratory depression.

Treatment

Analgesics such as morphine, buprenorphine or pentazocine should be administered as necessary (Table 2.4). The respiratory depression caused by such analgesics is more than adequately compensated for by the improved tidal volume that results from the patient breathing more comfortably.

The pneumothorax or haemothorax should then be treated by thoracocentesis.

DIAPHRAGMATIC RUPTURE (Table 2.5)

Traumatic rupture of the diaphragm is a potential sequel of penetrating and blunt injury, the site and extent of the tear

Table 2.4 Opiate analgesics suitable for use in the dog and cat.

Drug	Dose (dog)	Dose (cat)
Morphine sulphate	0.2 mg/kg (maximum 15 mg)	0.1 mg/kg (maximum 1 mg)
Pethidine hydrochloride	2 mg/kg	2 mg/kg (maximum 10 mg)
Buprenorphine	0.01 mg/kg	0.01–0.03 mg/kg
Pentazocine	1–2 mg/kg	1–2 mg/kg

dictating the severity of the condition. This may range from
sudden death, owing to massive lung collapse or rupture of
a major vessel, to less severe cases where a lobe of the liver,
the stomach or some of the small intestines move into the
thorax. The resultant respiratory distress may be aggravated
by changes in posture or by feeding. In the case of a left-
sided rupture the stomach almost invariably moves into the
chest and this generally involves some degree of torsion (Fig.
2.7). Thus left-sided ruptures may be complicated at any time,
and with great rapidity, by gastric dilation. In the right-sided
rupture the liver invariably enters the chest and is often
accompanied by a partial torsion of the posterior vena cava.
This may result in intrathoracic transudate formation and
further collapse of the lung tissue.

Diaphragmatic rupture in the cat is frequently in the midline
so that both pleural cavities are involved. Conversely, in the
dog the injury generally only involves one hemithorax.
Neverthless cats appear to be remarkably resistant to this
injury and survive the most extensive trauma with incredible
fortitude.

Table 2.5 Signs of diaphragmatic rupture.

Dyspnoea
Solid viscera within the chest may result in:

  muffled or displaced heart sounds
  displacement of the apex beat
  intestinal borborygmi
  areas of reduced resonance
  increased resonance in areas of trapped loops of bowel/stomach

Diaphragmatic rupture should be confirmed radiographically. Common
signs include:

  loss of the diaphragm line
  the presence of abdominal organs within the thorax and/or the
    absence of such organs within the abdomen
  the presence of gas filled loops of bowel within the chest
  displacement of the cardiac silhouette
  the presence of pleural fluid

In doubtful cases the position of the stomach and small intestines can
readily be checked by contrast radiography using 100% w/v barium
sulphate (8–12 ml/kg bodyweight)

Treatment

The diaphragmatic tear should be repaired under general anaesthesia with intermittent positive pressure ventilation. Unless there is severe respiratory distress repair can be delayed until the patient is in a reasonable state to undergo general anaesthesia. The presence of a gas-filled distended stomach or an incarcerated abdominal organ is the common reason for such distress and both conditions require immediate correction.

Anaesthesia must be induced with the minimum of stress to the animal. Struggling should be avoided and it is helpful to pre-oxygenate with a loose-fitting face mask using a flow rate of 3–4 litres/min. This is done with the patient in sternal recumbency to avoid altering the position of the trapped viscera within the chest, thereby collapsing yet more lung parenchyma. The surgeon should scrub up before the induction of anaesthesia in order that no time is lost in relieving the condition.

A ventral midline laparotomy provides good access to both sides of the chest and permits inspection of the abdominal viscera. It may be necessary to enlarge the tear in order that the trapped viscera can be returned safely to the abdomen. The edges of the tear should be coapted with horizontal mattress sutures of polyglycolic acid (Dexon; Davies & Geck) or polyglactin 910 (Vicryl; Ethicon).

Postoperative drainage of the chest is always advisable. Even when there is no obvious evidence of pulmonary damage the temptation to eliminate the surgical pneumothorax by "laying" the last suture in the diaphragmatic closure and then holding the lungs in full expansion while the suture is tied should be resisted. The repair of the tear in the diaphragm is not airtight and during the time that it takes to close the abdomen air will enter the chest. Even after closure, the pneumoperitoneum may be slowly sucked through the diaphragmatic defect into the thorax, adding yet further to the respiratory inefficiency.

The possibility of adhesions must be borne in mind in longstanding cases but rarely do they present any real surgical problem. There is, however, potential danger in reinflating lung tissue that has been collapsed for a long period of time as this may lead to pulmonary oedema. It is preferable to

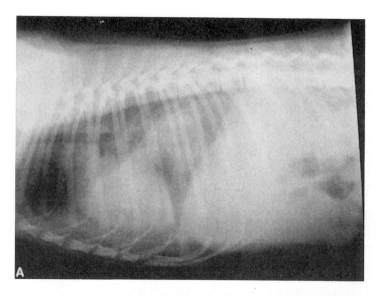

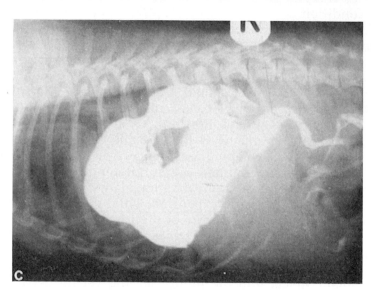

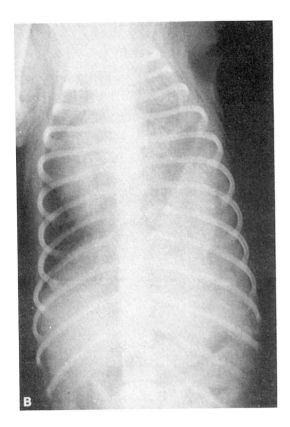

Fig. 2.7
Lateral (A) and dorsoventral (B)
projections of the thorax of a
Cavalier King Charles spaniel.
There is an increased soft tissue
density in the caudal chest with
anterior displacement of the left
caudal lung lobe. The heart is
displaced to the right. Pleural fluid
is evident in the left hemithorax.
(C) Following the administration of
barium sulphate the position of the
stomach can be seen clearly
within the chest. The case was
diagnosed as left-sided
diaphragmatic rupture.

encourage re-expansion by draining the chest after surgery
rather than by overzealously inflating the lungs while repairing
the diaphragmatic tear.

DAMAGE TO THE LUNG PARENCHYMA

Pulmonary contusion (Table 2.6)

Pulmonary contusion is caused by rapid compression–
decompression forces to the chest wall or airways. Intrapulmonary haemorrhage readily clots within the spongy pulmonary parenchyma and its clinical significance depends upon
the volume of the tissue involved (Fig. 2.8).

Table 2.6 Signs of pulmonary contusion.

Tachypnoea and dyspnoea
± Haemoptysis
Râles or silent areas on auscultation

Pulmonary contusion appears radiographically as areas of variable patchy density with an alveolar pattern

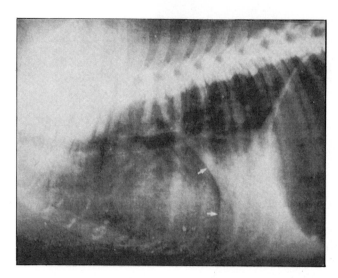

Fig. 2.8
Lateral projection of the thorax of a chow. There is a widespread alveolar pattern with patchy ill-defined densities. A pleural line is evident between the middle and caudal lobes (arrowed). Widespread pulmonary haemorrhage was diagnosed.

Treatment

Broad spectrum antibiotics should be administered as prophylaxis against pneumonia in the damaged lung parenchyma (eg, ampicillin or potentiated sulphonamides). Aspirate the trachea if there is a significant accumulation of secretions or haemorrhage.

Laceration of the lung (Table 2.7)

Laceration of the lung may occur by penetrating injuries or by violent compression forces, with or without fracture of the ribs.

Table 2.7 Signs of lung laceration.

See signs of:

 pulmonary contusion
 pneumothorax
 haemothorax

Treatment

Continuous thoracocentesis should be employed until the leak seals. With severe damage a persistent leak of blood and air is evident. While this is suggestive of a lacerated lung it is not possible to confirm without recourse to a thoracotomy.

Depending upon the extent of the laceration either a lobectomy should be carried out or the damaged portion should be resected. The undamaged tissue is oversewn with 3/0 chromic catgut on an atraumatic needle using the Parker–Kerr technique developed for oversewing bowel.

DISRUPTION OF THE AIRWAYS

The trachea and bronchi can be damaged by penetrating or non-penetrating trauma. Probably the commonest cause of dyspnoea following trauma is the condition of pneumothorax (Fig. 2.9 and Table 2.8). This is caused by air entering the pleural cavity and causing a concomitant collapse of lung tissue. No matter how slight, this collapse gives rise to a venous-arterial shunt and the raised intrapleural pressure impairs venous return to the heart. The end result is a decrease in arterial oxygen tension.

Simple pneumothorax

In the majority of cases the leak is caused by sudden non-penetrating trauma to the chest wall which momentarily raises the intrathoracic pressure. If this occurs against a closed glottis then alveolar tissue may rupture. In many cases the leak will be small but in others sufficient air will enter the pleural cavity to cause marked dyspnoea.

38   *J. E. F. Houlton*

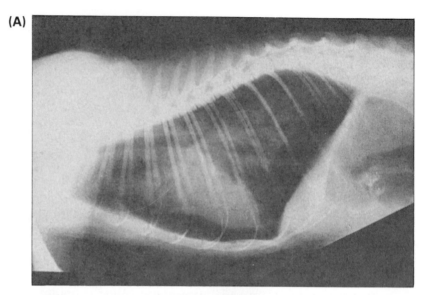

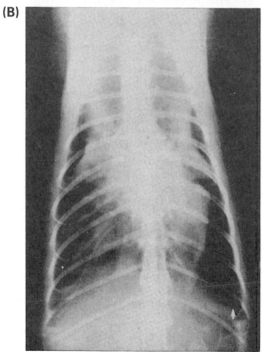

Fig. 2.9
Lateral (A) and dorsoventral (B)
projections of a cat's thorax. The
cardiac silhouette is elevated from the
sternum and there is evidence of free
pleural air in both hemithoraces. This
is particularly evident on the left side
with collapse of the lung lobes and
rounding of the costophrenic angle
(arrowed). Bilateral pneumothorax was
diagnosed.

Table 2.8 Signs of pneumothorax.

Dyspnoea—mild to moderate in simple cases
  —severe in open and tension pneumothoraces
Absence of respiratory sounds in affected part of the chest
Orthopnoea (a fixed hyperexpanded chest)
Chest wound(s)—open pneumothorax
Hyper-resonance of chest
Muffled heart sounds

Radiographic examination may be necessary to identify mild cases of simple pneumothorax. More severely affected patients are obviously dyspnoeic but they still require radiography to confirm the cause. Signs include separation of the cardiac silhouette from the sternum in the recumbent lateral projection and an absence of vascular shadows at the periphery of the lung fields in the dorsoventral projection

A traumatic pneumothorax often results from a road traffic accident or it may be seen in the coursing greyhound or whippet falling over at speed.

Open pneumothorax

A dramatic form of pneumothorax is caused by a penetrating wound of the chest wall. This results in an immediate and total collapse of the lung on the affected side and air can be heard entering the chest wound at each respiratory effort—the so-called open sucking pneumothorax. Besides the immediate acute effect of complete unilateral lung collapse there is also the insidious effect of the paradoxical respiration which exists all the time the chest wound is open.

Tension pneumothorax

A tension pneumothorax may develop with an open pneumo-thorax or when a small bronchus ruptures and pleural tissue acts as a one-way valve, ie, air accumulates in the pleural space during inspiration but is not expelled during expiration. The profound respiratory effort caused by the massive release of free air into the pleural cavity merely pumps yet more air from the bronchial tree into the pleural space, thus aggravating the situation and raising the intrapleural pressure above atmospheric pressure. The presence of air under tension in one hemithorax causes the mobile mediastinum to be displaced from the midline, thereby partially collapsing the remaining functional lung and adding yet further to the respiratory embarrassment.

Treatment of pneumothorax

First, assess the degree of pneumothorax. If the animal is not unduly dyspnoeic breathing room air, cage rest is appropriate. Monitor the degree of dyspnoea and be prepared for aspiration should the animal deteriorate.

Intermittent or continuous drainage should be instituted if the rate of leakage is sufficient to cause continued distress. However, if continuous suction over 48 h fails to seal the breach, a thoracotomy to surgically repair it should be considered. *A tension pneumothorax requires immediate thoraco-centesis to preserve the animal's life.*

Subcutaneous emphysema (Table 2.9, Figs 2.10 and 2.11)

A less serious, yet nonetheless spectacular condition may arise from rupture of the lung tissue near the hilus of the lung. Instead of entering the pleural cavity the released air tracks along the interstitial connective tissue of the bronchial tree down to the hilus where it enters the mediastinum. The air then dissects its way along the mediastinum and collects in the subcutaneous connective tissue of the neck and face.

Table 2.9 Signs of subcutaneous emphysema.

Subcutaneous emphysema of neck and head

The presence of air within the mediastinum and the subcutaneous tissues can be confirmed radiographically. The presence of a pneumomediastinum is best seen on a lateral projection of the chest when the air, acting as a negative contrast agent, provides a clear outline of the cranial mediastinal vessels and of the walls of the oesophagus and trachea

---

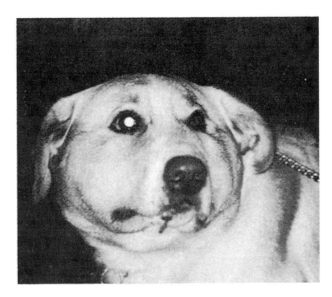

Fig. 2.10
Subcutaneous
emphysema of the
neck and face of a
crossbred labrador
with a pneumo-
mediastinum.

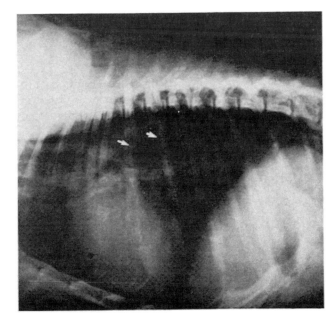

Fig. 2.11
Lateral projection of
the thorax of a
spaniel. Note the rib
fractures (arrowed)
and the
subcutaneous
emphysema. A
pneumomediastinum
is present, outlining
the structures of the
cranial mediastinum,
and a pneumo-
retroperitoneum
outlines the right
kidney. The
conditions and
lesions diagnosed
included rib
fractures,
subcutaneous
emphysema,
pneumomediastinum
and
pneumoretroperitoneum.

The condition is rarely dangerous although the emphysema may take days or weeks to resolve.

Treatment

First, other traumatic causes of pneumomediastinum, such as deep wounds of the neck, tracheobronchial leaks (respiratory distress is generally rapid and severe) or oesophageal ruptures, should be checked for. If none of these are present treatment is not generally required.

DAMAGE TO THE HEART AND VESSELS

Cardiac tamponade (Table 2.10)

Rupture of the cardiac chambers or laceration of the coronary vessels causes cardiac tamponade providing the pericardium is intact. This prevents adequate cardiac filling, particularly of the right ventricle, which results in reduced venous return and causes a dramatic drop in the cardiac output.

Treatment

In theory the pericardium can be opened and the source of haemorrhage identified. The epicardium and myocardium may be sutured and a lacerated coronary vessel can be ligated either side of the tear. In practice the lesion is rarely identified let alone treated.

Table 2.10 Signs of cardiac tamponade.

Muffling of the heart sounds
Loss of the apex beat
Congestion of the superficial veins
Weak thready pulse

The diagnosis can be difficult to confirm and it may be necessary to perform pericardiocentesis

Haemothorax (Table 2.11)

Crushing trauma may rupture the myocardium, pericardium or the major vessels of the cranial mediastinum. A massive haemothorax ensues and death is generally rapid. A less dramatic form of haemothorax follows rupture of the smaller vessels such as occurs in lacerations of the lung and chest wall.

Treatment

Thoracocentesis should be performed and intravenous fluid therapy instituted if hypovolaemic shock is imminent. If severe bleeding continues surgical exploration should be considered.

Myocardial contusions (Fig. 2.12, Table 2.12)

Contusions of the myocardium may result in post traumatic dysrhythmias, although it may be 12–24 h before these are

Table 2.11 Signs of haemothorax.

Dyspnoea
Dullness on percussion
Muffled cardiac and, or, respiratory sounds

Radiographic examination of the patient with free intrapleural fluid must be performed with care. It is important not to roll the animal into dorsal recumbency since the caudal lobes may suddenly collapse as a result of the redistribution of the fluid. This causes severe respiratory embarrassment and may even be fatal.

Radiographic signs of free pleural fluid include:

collapse of lung lobes with scalloped margins
"fissuring", ie, the presence of a soft tissue density between adjacent lobes
a soft tissue density between lung margins and the thoracic wall

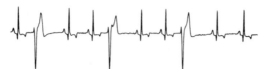

Fig. 2.12
ECG signs of myocardial contusions.
Lead II tracing showing premature
ventricular contractions at the second,
fifth and eighth complexes.

Table 2.12 Signs of myocardial contusions.

Irregular heart rhythm
Irregular pulse strength and rhythm
ECG changes

apparent. The most frequent changes are premature ventricular contractions and altered ST segments.

Treatment

Specific treatment is not usually required as the condition resolves with resolution of the primary cause.

DAMAGE TO THE OESOPHAGUS (Table 2.13)

Traumatic damage to the oesophagus is rare and is usually the result of perforating injuries from within the lumen. These

Table 2.13 Signs of oesophageal damage (Figs. 2.13 and 2.14).

Dyspnoea
Pain
Dysphagia
Ptyalism (excessive salivation)

The lesion should be suspected if an unexpected pneumomediastinum is detected radiographically. Other radiographic signs include evidence of mediastinal or pleural fluid.

The diagnosis is confirmed by oesophagoscopy or contrast radiography of the oesophagus using a non-ionic water-soluble compound such as iohexol (Omnipaque; Nyegaard)

provoke an intense mediastinitis and, as leakage of the oesophageal contents continues, a pyothorax may develop.

Treatment

A thoracotomy should be performed in order to debride and surgically repair the oesophageal tear. Daily lavage, with normal saline and metronidazole (Torgyl; May & Baker) via a thoracic drainage tube, will reduce the pleural contamination and combat anaerobic organisms. A giving set attached to the drainage tube can be used both to introduce and to drain the lavaging solution. The fluid is initially introduced under gravity; the animal is then stood on a table and the empty bag placed on the floor. The bag will refill and the possibility of an iatrogenic pneumothorax will be reduced.

Broad spectrum antibiosis (ampicillin or potentiated sulphonamides) should be instituted. Ampicillin may also be added to the lavaging solution.

Food should not be given by mouth for 3–5 days; instead provide fluids and calories by intravenous therapy.

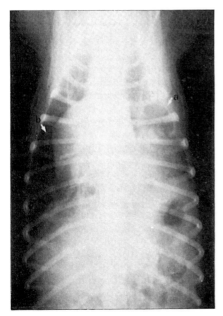

Fig. 2.13
Dorsoventral projection of the thorax of a retriever. Note the pleural fluid on the left side (a) and the fissure on the right (b). Bilateral pleural fluid was diagnosed.

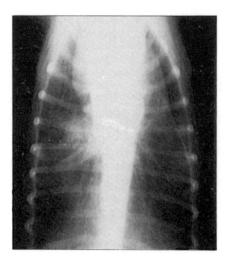

Fig. 2.14
Dorsoventral projection of the thorax of a German
shepherd dog. There is bilateral fissuring. The
mediastinum is widened and denser than normal.
Mediastinal and pleural fluid was diagnosed.

CONCLUSIONS

A systematic evaluation of the patient should identify those
conditions requiring immediate surgery. Fortunately these are
not as common as the less dramatic conditions which
should respond to conservative treatment. However, regular
monitoring of the patient's condition is essential and the
clinician must always be prepared to adopt a more aggressive
approach.

FURTHER READING

Kagan, K. G. (1980) *Veterinary Clinics of North America* **10**, 641.
Kirk, R. W. & Bistner, S. I. (1981) *Handbook of Veterinary Procedures and
    Emergency Treatment*. Philadelphia, W. B. Saunders.
Kolata, R. J. (1981) *Veterinary Clinics of North America* **11**, 103.
Sherding, R. G. (1985) *Medical Emergencies*. Edinburgh, Churchill Liv-
    ingstone.

CHAPTER 3

Acute Trauma in Small Animals 3: Orthopaedic Injuries

HAMISH DENNY

INTRODUCTION

A protocol for the initial assessment and management of the acute trauma case has already been described in Chapter 1. Wounds, fractures and dislocations are usually obvious on clinical examination and there is a natural tendency to concentrate on these and miss the more serious internal injuries. The general and local priorities for assessment and management are given in Table 3.1.

Table 3.1 Priorities for assessment and management of orthopaedic injuries.

General priorities	Local priorities
Maintain an airway	Head injuries
Maintain blood volume	Chest injury
Relieve pain	Abdominal injury
	Spinal injury
	Orthopaedic injury

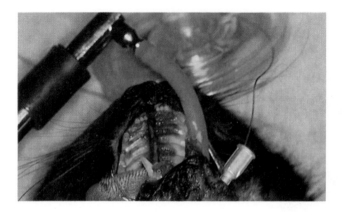

Fig. 3.1
A number 16 needle
is used as a guide to
pass a length of
orthopaedic wire
around the
mandibular
symphysis just
caudal to the canine
teeth.

HEAD INJURY

Upper airway obstruction can occur in the animal with
fractures of the mandible and/or maxilla, particularly if it is
concussed, because blood and mucus tend to accumulate in
the back of the pharynx. It is important to remove this material
and, if necessary, pass an endotracheal tube to maintain the
airway. Fracture of the mandibular symphysis is the most
common jaw fracture in the dog and cat and a simple method
of inserting a cerclage wire for fixation is illustrated here (Figs
3.1 and 3.2). In the cat, the injury may be complicated by
fracture of the hard palate (Fig. 3.3) and a tension band wire
placed between the carnassial teeth provides good stability
(Fig. 3.4).

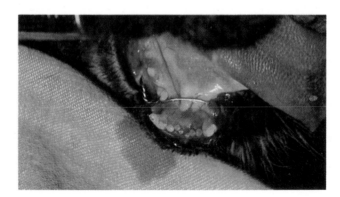

Fig. 3.2
The cerclage wire
has been tightened
compressing the
symphysis.

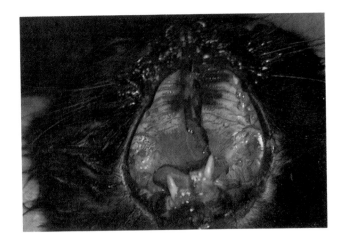

Fig. 3.3
Cat with fractures of
the hard palate and
mandibular
symphysis.

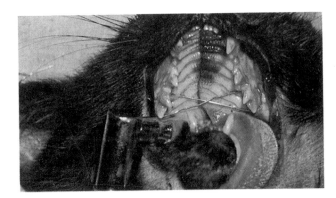

Fig. 3.4
The two halves of the
hard palate have
been apposed and
stabilized using a
tension band wire
placed between the
roots of the
carnassial teeth.

Fractures of the neurocranium may be associated with brain damage, either directly or indirectly through haemorrhage into the cranial vault. Few cases are presented for treatment presumably because the injury is often fatal. Associated signs will, of course, vary with the degree and location of the brain damage. Linear fractures may require no treatment except the administration of corticosteroids (betamethasone or dexamethasone, 2–4 mg/kg/day) to control oedema. Mannitol should not be used for the control of oedema except during or after surgery as it may potentiate further haemorrhage.

Intracranial haemorrhage and oedema may be associated with:

(a) Loss of consciousness
(b) Dilatation of one or both pupils or other evidence of cranial nerve injury
(c) Motor dysfunction such as hemiparesis or decerebrate rigidity.

If any of these signs are present and progressive, then cranial decompression should be considered as an emergency procedure.

SPINAL INJURY

Acute trauma to the spinal cord results from fractures, dislocations, disc protrusions or concussion. Fractures and/or dislocations of the spine occur most frequently in the terminal thoracic region. The injury generally causes paraplegia and the prognosis for recovery is poor unless there is still deep pain sensation in the hindlimbs. Plain radiography is the most useful way of differentiating traumatic lesions of the cord (Fig. 3.5). There will be negative findings if trauma to the cord is due to concussion (spinal haemorrhage).

When there has been acute trauma to the spinal cord, treatment must be initiated within a few hours to be of benefit. Betamethasone or dexamethasone are given twice daily for 72 hours (total daily dose 2–4 mg/kg) and then gradually reduced. Decompression of the spinal cord by laminectomy is indicated if there is vertebral displacement or an explosive disc protrusion. Vertebral stability can be restored using a U-shaped pin and wire sutures (Gage 1971) (Fig. 3.6). Ideally surgery should be undertaken within 6 h of the accident and corticosteroids should be given to reduce cord oedema.

Fractures in the cervical region most frequently involve the atlas and axis. Although there may be considerable displacement of fractures of the cranial cervical vertebrae, the resultant neurological deficits are often remarkably mild. The main presenting sign is cervical pain. The prognosis is good and the majority of cases will recover with conservative

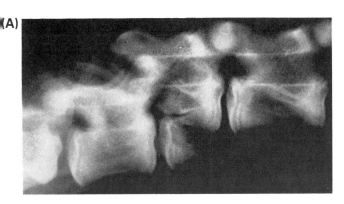

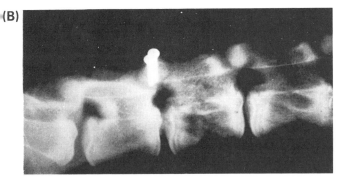

Fig. 3.5
(A) Lateral radiograph showing fracture of the centrum of L6 with dislocation of the articular facets between L6/7, in a six-month-old male German shepherd dog. (B) Radiograph taken after surgical reduction and immobilization with two screws through the articular facets. The dog recovered within six weeks of surgery and had no further problems during a one year follow up period. (Reproduced from Denny and others (1982) with permission of the editor of the *Journal of Small Animal Practice.*)

treatment. Dogs with undisplaced fractures are given strict rest for four weeks while those with displaced or unstable fractures have the neck immobilized in a cast for four weeks.

Fractures of the caudal three lumbar vertebrae may compress the cauda equina causing intense pain, paresis or paraplegia, with urinary retention in some cases. There is plenty of room for the cauda equina within the neural canal and considerable vertebral displacement can be tolerated without necessarily causing permanent neurological dysfunction. Decompressive laminectomy is generally unnecessary but reduction and fixation of the fracture/dislocation should be undertaken to relieve pain. The prognosis is reasonably good except for cases with lumbosacral dislocation. Here the dog regains the use of its hindlegs but bladder paralysis persists.

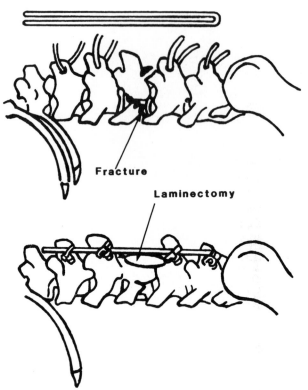

Fig. 3.6
U-shaped pin and wire
sutures used to stabilize
a lumbar vertebral
fracture.

ORTHOPAEDIC INJURIES—EXAMINATION

The common traumatic conditions of the fore- and hindlimbs are summarized in Tables 3.2 and 3.3.

Dislocations and ligamentous ruptures tend to be seen in mature dogs over one year of age. The same trauma in immature animals is more likely to cause a fracture or separation of an epiphysis. Orthopaedic injuries alone are seldom life-threatening unless they are associated with gross haemorrhage. (A soft tissue swelling the size of a clenched fist around a fracture site is equivalent to approximately 750 ml blood.) However, chest injuries, particularly pneumothorax, are common complications of fractures of the humerus and scapula. In all road traffic accident cases, a careful clinical and radiological examination should be done to check for chest

Table 3.2 Traumatic conditions of the forelimb.

Scapular fractures
Surgical treatment is required for:

(a) intra-articular fractures
(b) avulsion fractures
(c) displaced fractures of scapular neck

Other fractures can be managed conservatively

Shoulder dislocations
Gross instability with lateral dislocation of humeral head most often

Humeral shaft fractures
Distal third mainly, spiral or oblique, often comminuted

Elbow

(a) Dislocation
      Radial head dislocates laterally, forearm swung out laterally, held
      forward and supinated
(b) Condylar fractures
      Spaniels are particularly prone to this injury. Lateral condyle
      fractures most frequently

(c) Fracture of the olecranon

Shaft fractures of radius and ulna
Generally transverse and involve distal third

Carpus

(a) Fracture of accessory carpal bone
(b) Hyperextension of carpus due to rupture of plantar ligaments
(c) Dislocation

Metacarpus
Fractures and crush injuries common

Greyhound toe injuries

(a) Interphalangeal subluxations and dislocations
(b) Fractures of phalanges and sesamoids
(c) "Knocked up toe"

injuries, which should be treated before embarking on fracture fixation. Many chest injuries are missed out on clinical examination but picked up on radiography. Cases with tension pneumothorax or intrapulmonary haemorrhage are obviously

Table 3.3 Traumatic conditions of the hindleg.

Pelvis
Fracture. Indications for surgical treatment: displaced fractures of
  weightbearing areas

(a)   Acetabulum
(b)   Ilium
(c)   Sacroiliac joint

Hip
(a)   Acetabular fractures
(b)   Fractures of the femoral head or neck ± trochanteric fractures
(c)   Dislocations

Femur
(a)   Fractures of the proximal femur
(b)   Fractures of the shaft
(c)   Supracondylar and condylar fractures

Stifle
(a)   Rupture of:
      anterior cruciate ligament ± damage to medial meniscus
      collateral ligament
      straight patellar ligament
(b)   Dislocation of the patella
(c)   Dislocation of the stifle
(d)   Avulsion of the tendon of origin of the long digital extensor muscle
(e)   Fractures of the distal femur (see above)
(f)   Fractures of the patella
(g)   Fractures of the proximal tibia,
      avulsion of the tibial crest,
      separation of the proximal epiphyses of the tibia

Tibia
(a)   Fractures of the proximal tibia (see above)
(b)   Fractures of the shaft
(c)   Distal tibial fractures
      (i) malleolar fractures
      (ii) separation of distal epiphysis

Hock
(a)   Malleolar fracture   ⎫ Dislocation of
(b)   Rupture of the collateral ligaments   ⎬ the tibiotarsal
(c)   Severe abrasion injury   ⎭ joint
(d)   Fractures of the os calcis
(e)   Injuries of the Achilles tendon
(f)   Intertarsal subluxation (rupture of plantar ligaments) (shelties, collies)
(g)   Fracture of the central tarsal bone
(h)   Fractures of the metatarsus and digits

an anaesthetic risk and surgery should be delayed (usually a matter of days) until resolution occurs. Nitrous oxide will rapidly increase the volume of a pneumothorax and should be avoided in the anaesthesia of such cases.

A serious potential complication of pelvic fracture is rupture of the bladder or urethra. Fortunately, this type of injury is uncommon. In a review of 123 pelvic fracture cases (Denny 1978), only one had bladder rupture and two had rupture of the urethra. Nevertheless, if there is any doubt about the integrity of the bladder or urethra, then cystography and/or urethrography should be undertaken.

It is beyond the scope of this paper to present the specific clinical features of individual fractures and dislocations. Radiography is essential to confirm the diagnosis and it is important, especially in fractures, to obtain both an anteroposterior and a lateral view of the lesion.

BASIC MANAGEMENT OF DISLOCATIONS

In all dislocations, reduction should be undertaken as soon as possible after the accident, preferably within 24 h. After reduction of a hip dislocation, the leg should be strapped in flexion, using an Ehmer sling (Fig. 3.7) for five days.

In cases of shoulder luxation, a body cast (Fig. 3.8) is applied for three weeks to prevent redislocation. The elbow, by contrast, requires little external support as good stability is restored immediately following reduction in most cases.

FIRST AID PROCEDURES FOR TEMPORARY IMMOBILIZATION OF FRACTURES OR INJURED JOINTS

ROBERT JONES BANDAGE (Fig. 3.9)

The Robert Jones bandage is a thick cotton wool bandage which acts as a splint and controls oedema. For these reasons, it is useful not only as a first aid measure for the temporary immobilization of fractures but also as a postoperative bandage for fractures which have been treated surgically. The bandage

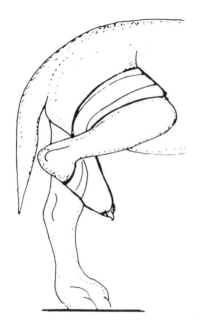

Fig. 3.7
Ehmer sling.

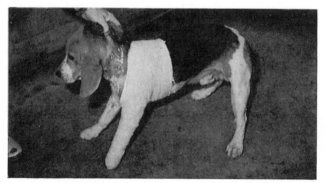

Fig. 3.8
Body cast.

is comfortable to wear and is generally well tolerated despite its bulk.

THOMAS EXTENSION SPLINT (Fig. 3.10)

Although this splint can be used as the sole method of fixation for stable fractures below the elbow or stifle, it is generally used only as a temporary splint for limb bone fractures. The

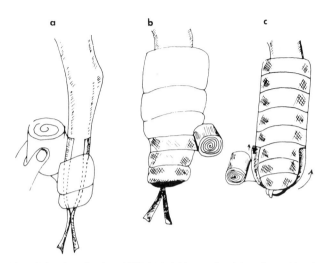

Fig. 3.9 Applying a Robert Jones bandage. (a) Elastoplast strips are placed down the cranial and caudal aspect of the foot (these will prevent the bandage slipping off the leg) and can be used for traction during application of the cotton wool layers. (b) A 1lb roll of cotton wool is split into two narrower ½ lb rolls and these are used to pad the leg. The total amount of cotton wool required ranges from ½ to 2 lb depending on the size of the dog. (c) The ends of the Elastoplast tape are flapped back to reveal the pads of the foot and then attached to the end of the bandage using Elastoplast. The cotton wool is tightly compressed with an Elastoplast bandage. (Reproduced from Denny, H. R. (1985) *A Guide to Canine Orthopaedic Surgery.* Oxford, Blackwell, with permission.)

splint is usually constructed from an aluminium rod, but coat hanger wire can be used in small dogs. A ring is made in the rod to fit around the base of the leg. The base of the ring is bent in at an angle to avoid pressure on the femoral blood vessels and the ring is padded with cotton wool. The splint is pushed firmly into the inguinal region and the cranial bar of the splint is bent to conform to the leg's normal angulation in the standing position. Elastoplast strips are used to fix the foot to the end of the bar. The upper part of the leg is also attached to the cranial bar with Elastoplast, while a thick band of Elastoplast is placed round both bars and the hock.

VELPEAU SLING BANDAGE

This bandage is used to immobilize shoulder and scapular injuries and to prevent weightbearing. A conforming gauze bandage is wrapped around the paw, the leg is flexed and the bandage is brought up over the lateral aspect of the

(A)   **(B)**   **(C)**

(D)   **(E)**

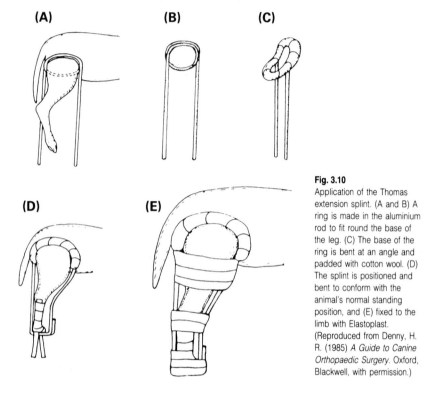

Fig. 3.10
Application of the Thomas extension splint. (A and B) A ring is made in the aluminium rod to fit round the base of the leg. (C) The base of the ring is bent at an angle and padded with cotton wool. (D) The splint is positioned and bent to conform with the animal's normal standing position, and (E) fixed to the limb with Elastoplast. (Reproduced from Denny, H. R. (1985) *A Guide to Canine Orthopaedic Surgery.* Oxford, Blackwell, with permission.)

shoulder and around the chest. Several layers are applied and then covered with Elastoplast.

THE APPROPRIATE METHOD OF FRACTURE FIXATION

CLOSED REDUCTION AND EXTERNAL FIXATION (Fig. 3.11)

Closed reduction and external fixation with casts or splints should be reserved for stable shaft fractures, ie, greenstick, transverse and blunt oblique fractures. At least 50% of the fracture surfaces should be in contact and it is important to immobilize the joint above and below the fracture. The method is limited to fractures distal to the elbow and stifle.

OPEN REDUCTION AND INTERNAL FIXATION
(Fig. 3.12)

The management of long bone fractures differs according to the anatomical location of the fracture and the age and species of animal. There are four basic sites of fracture and each is managed in a specific way.

Avulsion fractures

Avulsion fractures of, for example, the olecranon, greater trochanter, patella, tibial crest and os calcis, are all fractures in which the fragment is distracted by the tensile force of the muscle, tendon or ligament which inserts on the fragment. Initial fixation is achieved with Kirschner wires or a lag screw used in combination with a tension band wire (18 or 20 gauge) to counteract the tensile force acting on the fragment.

Articular fractures

With articular fractures, for example, of the lateral condyle of the humerus, open reduction is essential to allow accurate anatomical reconstruction of the joint surfaces. Fixation is achieved with a transcondylar lag screw and a Kirschner wire to prevent rotation.

Shaft fractures

Shaft fractures can be broadly divided into stable and unstable fractures.

Stable fractures are the transverse, blunt oblique or greenstick fractures in which fragments interlock and resist shortening. The only fixation necessary is to prevent angular deformity and, depending on site, this may be done with either a cast, intramedullary pin or plate.

The unstable fractures are oblique, spiral or comminuted. The fragments do not interlock. The method of fixation should maintain length of the bone and prevent angulation and rotation. The ideal way of doing this is to reconstruct the

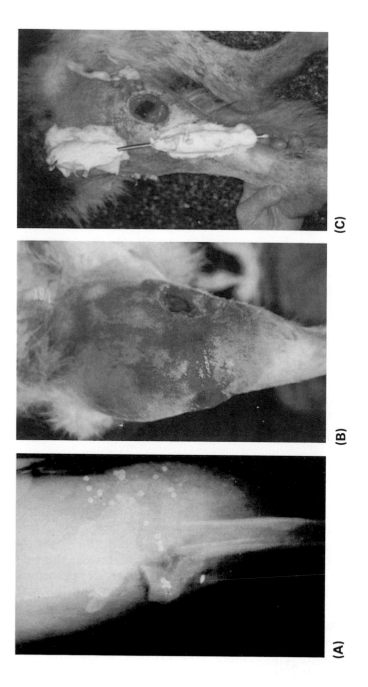

(A)   (B)   (C)

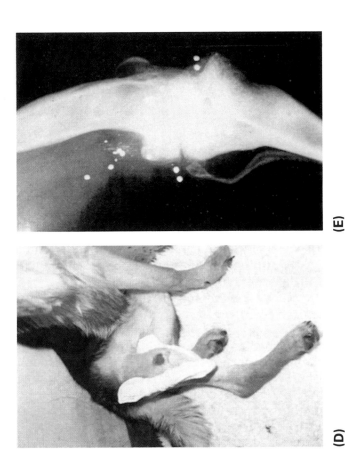

(D)

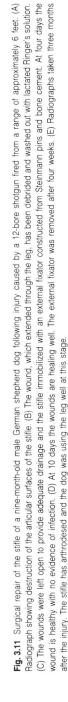

(E)

Fig. 3.11 Surgical repair of the stifle of a nine-month-old male German shepherd dog following injury caused by a 12-bore shotgun fired from a range of approximately 6 feet. (A) Radiograph showing destruction of the articular surfaces of the stifle. (B) The wound, which extended through the leg, has been debrided and washed out with lactated Ringer's solution. (C) The wounds were left open to provide adequate drainage and the stifle immobilized with an external fixator constructed from Steinmann pins and bone cement. At four days the wound is healthy with no evidence of infection. (D) At 10 days the wounds are healing well. The external fixator was removed after four weeks. (E) Radiographs taken three months after the injury. The stifle has arthrodesed and the dog was using the leg well at this stage.

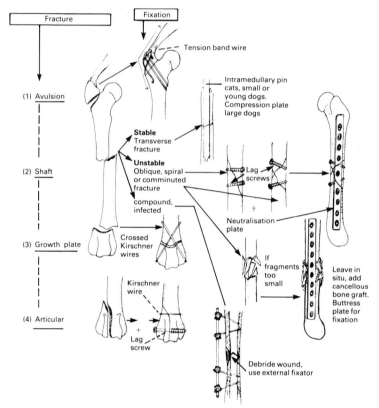

Fig. 3.12 Selection of appropriate method for fracture fixation.

bone with lag screws and apply a neutralization plate. If the fragments are too small for lag screw fixation, they are left *in situ* and a plate is applied to maintain bone length. In this situation, the plate functions as a buttress plate.

Shaft fractures of all long bones in the cat can usually be succesfully repaired using an intramedullary pin, either alone or in combination with cerclage wire in oblique or comminuted fractures. In the dog, the intramedullary pin should be reserved for stable fractures of the middle third of the femoral or humeral shaft. The pin should fit tightly within the medullary cavity to ensure adequate stability and, for this reason, the method is limited to small or young dogs. In larger dogs, especially those with humeral shaft fractures, a plate is the preferred method of treatment.

Although stable fractures of the radius and ulna or tibia are often successfully treated by the application of a cast, especially in puppies, compression plate fixation gives consistently good results and this method is recommended for displaced fractures in adult dogs.

In compound or infected shaft fractures, an external fixator is used to provide stability following thorough wound debridement.

Epiphyseal separations

Early open reduction should be carried out and Kirschner wires are used for fixation.

Timing of surgery

It is important to consider the soft tissue response to injury when considering the optimal time to carry out internal fixation of a fracture. The local circulation will be disturbed causing hypoxia, acidosis and oedema of the tissues, an ideal situation for infection to become established. Surgery should either be undertaken before the circulation becomes compromised, ideally within six hours (maximum 24 h), or it should be delayed for between 4–6 days to allow the circulation to the soft tissues to become re-established. Urgent surgical treatment is needed for articular fractures, growth plate fractures and compound fractures. Early surgery is also preferable for pelvic fractures and severely comminuted shaft fractures before muscle contracture makes reduction difficult.

If antibiotic prophylaxis is to be provided, high blood concentrations are established by intravenous injection one hour before surgery. A five-day course of treatment is given. Ampicillin is used most frequently. Poor asepsis, prolonged operating time and disruption of blood supply to the bone by rough handling of tissues and stripping periosteum or soft tissue attachments all predispose to infection. Antibiotic prophylaxis is no substitute for poor standards of asepsis and surgical technique.

REFERENCES

Denny, H. R. (1978) *Journal of Small Animal Practice* **19**, 151.
Denny, H. R., Gibbs, C. & Holt, P. E. (1982) *Journal of Small Animal Practice* **23**, 425.
Gage, E. D. (1971) *Veterinary Medicine/Small Animal Clinician* **66**, 295.

CHAPTER 4

Acute Trauma in Small Animals 4: Abdominal Injuries

HAROLD PEARSON

INTRODUCTION

Trauma may result in multiple injuries. The occurrence of soft tissue lesions may initially be overlooked because of more obvious orthopaedic problems.

TYPES OF ABDOMINAL TRAUMA

(1) Damage to the abdominal wall and diaphragm
(2) Damage to solid organs
(3) Damage to hollow viscera

ABDOMINAL WALL AND DIAPHRAGM

In both dogs and cats rupture of the diaphragm is a common sequel of trauma. It often accompanies orthopaedic injuries and diaphragmatic integrity should be radiographically checked as a routine in such cases. In the dog, movement of the stomach into the pleural cavity is potentially rapidly fatal should gastric dilation occur. Radiographic evidence of a gastric shadow cranial to the diaphragm warrants immediate surgery to repair the rupture.

Rupture of the abdominal wall can be caused by traffic accidents, fights, and sometimes, closing doors. In both the dog and cat perforating abdominal wounds may be complicated by some degree of evisceration, especially of omentum.

Abdominal wall rupture is particularly common in the cat, often affecting the ventral abdomen, possibly with avulsion of prepubic attachments. During pregnancy such ruptures may result in gross displacement of the gravid uterus into a directly subcutaneous position. Ventral ruptures may initially be masked by local bruising, haemorrhage and oedema which can be left to subside before corrective surgery is undertaken. In cases of diffuse painful lesions which are difficult to examine by palpation, the integrity of the abdominal wall can be assessed by contrast gastrointestinal radiography.

Occasionally, "run on" stick injuries can have startling effects, the foreign body traversing both the thoracic and abdominal cavity through a perforated diaphragm before emerging from the body some distance from the point of entry. Sometimes there is no serious visceral damage whatsoever.

SOLID ORGAN TRAUMA

Solid viscera may be damaged by blunt trauma, penetrating abdominal or thoracic wounds, or gunshot injuries. On the whole, ballistic injuries are more likely to damage the muscular and skeletal tissues than abdominal viscera. Viscera which lie under the costal arch are protected to some degree. However, rupture of the liver is a common cause of fatal intraperitoneal bleeding. The kidneys are protected by the sublumbar muscles but bruising and perirenal retroperitoneal haemorrhage may cause haematuria, usually of a transient nature. The spleen is highly vulnerable to abdominal trauma and is often totally divided with consequent haemorrhage from each fragment.

Serious rupture of parenchymatous organs usually results in gross haemoperitoneum and associated signs of pallor, shock, localized pain and failing circulation. The presence of free intraperitoneal blood can be suspected on palpation and confirmed by paracentesis. The management of such cases requires careful assessment, with greater reliance on clinical signs than haematocrit values. Fluid replacement therapy, ideally with whole blood but otherwise with colloids or crystalloids, may improve and stabilize the patient's circulatory status.

Continuing clinical deterioration with a packed cell volume below 20% despite such therapy, justifies exploratory laparotomy. Splenic haemorrhage can then be stopped by total or partial splenectomy and localized hepatic bleeding controlled by lobectomy, but hepatic injuries often result in multiple fissures which are not amenable to surgical repair. The facilities for administering large quantities of blood continuously to such patients are not usually available in veterinary practices.

HOLLOW ORGAN RUPTURE

The urinary, biliary and intestinal tracts may also be perforated by trauma.

URINARY TRACT

The distended urinary bladder of the dog is highly vulnerable to rupture and its integrity should be checked by palpation or cystography in all cases of hind quarter trauma. Urethral ruptures are much less common but they occur particularly in association with pelvic fractures. In occasional cases, rupture of both urinary bladder and urethra may occur simultaneously.

Ureteric injuries are relatively rare but avulsion of one or both ureters, usually close to the kidney, may follow lumbar trauma in dogs or cats. The clinical signs of urinary tract rupture depend on the level of perforation. Rupture of the bladder allows urine to pass directly into the peritoneal cavity, with characteristic distension of the ventral abdomen within two or three days of the accident. It is important to realize, however, that such animals may continue to pass some urine down the urethra. Urination may continue with minor urethral tearing, but transection causes serious dysuria, sometimes with oedema-like fluid filling of soft tissues at the ischial arch and within the pelvic cavity. Bilateral ureteric avulsion also causes urine accumulation within the peritoneal cavity, but unilateral lesions are easily missed without excretion urography. Intraperitoneal accumulation of urine is associated with progressive abdominal distension, a fluid wave on percussion and systemic illness caused by worsening uraemia and other metabolic changes. The escape of urine on paracentesis confirms urinary tract rupture without localizing the site.

Urethral rupture may be suspected with pelvic fractures but retrograde urethrocystography is advisable in all patients with "urine ascites" in case both bladder and urethra are damaged. In the management of urinary tract rupture with free urine in the peritoneal cavity, it is most important to concentrate first on correcting metabolic changes before anaesthesia is induced for surgery. Uraemia, hyperkalaemia and metabolic acidosis can be assumed in such cases and preliminary fluid therapy is advisable to avoid the risk of death during or immediately after surgery.

Bladder tears are easily amenable to suture repair at laparotomy; in fact by the time surgery is performed the tear may be almost sealed by natural healing and local visceral adhesion. By contrast, urethral tears may prove impossible to repair.

Depending on the site, pelvic splitting may be necessary to allow attempted suturing of the tear over a catheter, but total transection may be associated with extensive local bleeding and gross separation of the urethral stumps. Insertion of an indwelling catheter as a stent may allow spontaneous healing but with the likelihood of subsequent stricture formation. An indwelling catheter is recommended after repair of both bladder and urethral tears but bladder lesions usually heal without complications. Ureteric tears or avulsion are treated by either suture repair (with subsequent risk of stricture) or ureteronephrectomy if the lesion is unilateral.

THE BILIARY TRACT

Biliary tract trauma is much less common than urinary rupture and it is largely confined to the dog. The injury results from penetrating wounds (often impalement) of the abdomen or thorax, or blunt trauma. The gall bladder, cystic and hepatic ducts and most commonly, the common bile duct may be affected.

Clinical signs are usually apparent within a few days but are sometimes not manifested for three or four weeks. Bile ascites, deepening icterus of mucous membranes, pale faeces, anorexia, vomiting and weight loss are associated with exceedingly high serum conjugated bilirubin and liver enzyme levels. The diagnosis is confirmed by aspiration of bile varying in colour from blackish green to deep yellow, on paracentesis. Cholangiography has proved unhelpful in diagnosis. The treatment is surgical, although there is evidence from failed suture repairs that biliary duct ruptures may heal spontaneously if the degree of bile ascites is controlled by periodic drainage.

In large, deep chested dogs, exposure of the biliary system at surgery requires wide abdominal retraction. Suction facilities or constant swabbing are necessary to allow identification of the rupture site. If the gall bladder is intact, it is gently squeezed (without emptying it) to watch for bile leakage in the duct system. In most cases the rupture affects the common bile duct, which may be perforated at more than one site.

Occasionally, leakage results from avulsion of the duct from the duodenum. Recent reviews of biliary tract surgery in the dog (Thompson 1981, Blass 1983) describe medical techniques such as T or Y tube stents and diverting biliary-enteric anastomoses for rupture repair. However, few veterinarians are practised in this aspect of surgery and simple suturing methods are preferable whenever possible.

Tears in the common bile duct are repaired with 4–0 silk on a non-cutting needle. Hepatic duct lesions are ligated on either side of the tear. If suture repair is impossible, salvage procedures such as cholecystectomy, cholecystoduodenostomy or cholecystojejunostomy may be attempted, provided, in the latter anastomotic procedures, that a stoma at least 2 cm diameter is created to prevent stricture formation and postoperative cholangitis.

Successful repair leads to rapid clinical improvement, but bile clearance from serosal and mucosal surfaces is much more gradual. Surgical failure is usually manifested within a few

days by gradual refilling of the peritoneal cavity; such cases
may be treated by continual abdominal drainage in the hope
that natural healing of the defect will occur. In medical terms,
a distinction is made between bile ascites and bile peritonitis
but this may not be valid for the dog. As with urine, it is
remarkable how little adverse effect, apart from discoloration,
results from free bile within the peritoneal cavity in dogs.

THE INTESTINAL TRACT

Damage to the gut may result from perforating abdominal
wounds, or intraluminal foreign bodies. The gut is also
vulnerable to the effects of blunt trauma. The latter type of
injury is not well documented but all reports indicate that its
clinical effects are insidious in onset, not always readily
recognizable in animals suffering from multiple injuries, and
rapidly fatal within even four days.
    Intestinal damage is attributed basically to the effect of
shearing between two apposing surfaces such as the abdominal
wall and the spine, and the presence of peritoneal fixed points
which appose certain intestinal segments to the spine. The
following pathological complications may ensue:

(1)   Mesenteric stripping, leading to segmental infarction
(2)   Mesenteric torsion, leading to vascular collapse
(3)   Mesenteric vessel thrombosis, leading to delayed infarction
(4)   Mesenteric or omental tearing, leading to intestinal
displacement and strangulation
(5)   Direct rupture of the bowel

All reports describe the development of the clinical signs
(Table 4.1).

Peritoneal lavage

The tentative diagnosis of intestinal injury is based on
clinical signs and radiographic evidence of peritonitis or
pneumoperitoneum from bowel rupture, delayed transit or
leakage of contrast agent or gross displacement of intestine,

Table 4.1 Development of clinical signs in gut injury.

Depression and pain on palpation
Presence of fresh blood in the rectum and faeces
Gradual accumulation of peritoneal fluid consisting of exudate and
  possibly bowel content
Tarry faeces
Firm, painful abdominal distension caused by peritonitis
Vomiting *but not in all cases*
Survival up to four days, although in some cases the clinical signs may
  be delayed for up to 10 days

probably with ileus. Bearing in mind the early fatality of such cases, immediate exploratory laparotomy might seem justified. However, as a means of avoiding unnecessary surgery, several authors have commented on the value of peritoneal lavage as a non-invasive method of diagnosing gut rupture or infarction.

After emptying the urinary bladder by catherization, a catheter of appropriate size is inserted, under local analgesia and with aseptic precautions, in the ventral abdomen. Escaping peritoneal fluid is collected for examination, and sterile saline solution, at the rate of 20 ml per kg bodyweight, is infused. The patient is gently rolled from side to side and the infused fluid is then harvested into a reservoir bottle by gently compressing the abdomen.

A crude method of assessing the returned fluid is to place a syringe with dark printing on its barrel under the tubing leading to the reservoir bottle. If the print can be read through the tube, regardless of the colour of the fluid, the result is considered negative, with no evidence of serious injury. If the printing cannot be read because of opacity of the fluid, serious abnormality can be inferred and the sample is subjected to the laboratory examinations given in Table 4.2.

It must be emphasized that paracentesis may yield apparently normal results despite the presence of extensive bowel infarction if the lesion is sequestrated within or outside the peritoneal cavity.

Kick and crush injuries to the abdomen may result in tearing of omenta or mesentery with subsequent gross displacement of stomach and/or intestine. Such cases show

Table 4.2 Laboratory examinations of peritoneal fluid.

Packed cell volume	After 500 ml infusion, every 1% packed cell volume means 10–20 ml of free blood in the peritoneal cavity
Sediment	Bacteria or vegetable fibres with neutrophils mean hollow viscus rupture
Bilirubin	Biliary or upper intestinal tract disruption
Amylase	Intestinal ischaemia or pancreatic damage
White blood cell count	More than 500/mm^3 indicates peritonitis Experimental inocula produce more than 1200/mm^3 within 3 h
Creatinine/urea	Levels more than those of serum imply urinary tract rupture

acute abdominal pain and may die very rapidly of shock before ischaemic change develops.

Most cases of serious intestinal injury require enterectomy and intensive supportive antibiotic and fluid therapy. Some are totally inoperable because of the extent of bowel infarction. Cases of simultaneous biliary and intestinal rupture are difficult to diagnose except by thorough exploration at laparotomy. The value of postoperative indwelling drainage/irrigation tubes is contentious. They may allow ascending infection of the peritoneal cavity and their efficacy can be impaired by adhesion of overlying omentum or mesentery.

REFERENCES AND FURTHER READING

Blass, C. E. (1983) *The Compendium of Continuing Education* **5**, 801.

Crane, S. W. (1980) *Veterinary Clinics of North America: Small Animal Practice* **10**, 655.

Crowe, D. T. & Crane, S. W. (1976) *Journal of the American Veterinary Medical Association* **168**, 700.

Dorn, S. A., Hufford, T. J. & Anderson, N. V. (1975) *Journal of the American Animal Hospital Association* **11**, 786.

Kolata, D. J. (1976) *Journal of the American Veterinary Medical Association* **168**, 697.

Kolata, D. J., Kraute, N. H. & Johnston, D. E. (1974) *Journal of the American Veterinary Medical Association* **164**, 499.

Schiller, A. G. (1975) *Proceedings of the 20th World Veterinary Congress, Thessalonika* **2**, 1659.
Thompson, S. M. R. (1981) *Journal of Small Animal Practice* **22**, 437.

CHAPTER 5

Free Skin Grafting in Small Animals

NICK MCGLENNON AND RICHARD WHITE

INTRODUCTION

A free skin graft (FSG) is an area of skin comprising both epidermis and varying depths of underlying dermis which is detached from a donor site and transferred to a recipient area. Because its original vascular supply is removed during harvesting, the graft's ultimate survival depends on the development of a new vascular supply from the recipient bed. By contrast a pedicle graft retains a vascular supply and its viability depends to a much lesser extent on the development of new capillaries. For most practical purposes free skin grafts are harvested from the same animal which is to receive the graft, ie, autografts.

WHAT ARE THE INDICATIONS FOR AN FSG?

Free skin grafts are useful in the reconstruction of any large cutaneous deficit. Properly applied and managed they can significantly reduce the time and expense that might be spent in managing a wound that is otherwise allowed to heal by epithelialization and contraction. They are particularly appropriate when dealing with lesions of the extremities (including digits) where the restricted availability of the skin often prohibits primary wound closure or the use of sliding or pedicle grafts. FSGs should be considered in the management of:

(1) Degloving injuries caused by automobile trauma
(2) Defects created by the excision of large neoplastic masses
(3) Burns

WHAT TYPE OF TISSUE WILL ACCEPT FSGs?

Broadly speaking there are three situations in which an FSG can be successfully applied:

(1) *A freshly created wound surface,* for example following the excision of a large cutaneous tumour (Fig. 5.1) or following the debridement of a lightly contaminated wound. The wound should be capable of providing sufficient vascular supply from the underlying tissue to support the graft. However, adequate haemostasis is essential prior to grafting to prevent haematomas developing under the graft which may interfere with graft "take".

It is important to bear in mind that any tissue in a fresh wound that has been deprived of its blood supply, eg, tendon stripped of its paratenon or bone which has lost its periosteum will *not* support an FSG. In such situations granulation tissue should be allowed to cover these tissues before grafting.

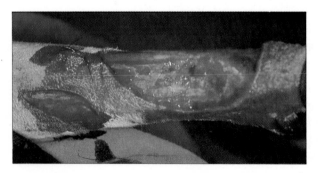

Fig. 5.1
Freshly created wound surface suitable for grafting following excision of a skin tumour.

(2) *Freshly granulating wounds,* for example following degloving or abrasion injuries. Before an FSG can be applied in these situations it is important to scrupulously debride the wound to remove as much contamination as possible (Fig. 5.2). This can be achieved by irrigation, surgical debridement, wet to dry dressings or by the use of chemical debridement, eg, Travase ointment (Flint Laboratories USA) or Dermisol (Beecham Animal Health) or by a combination of these methods. The process of debridement should be continued until fresh healthy, granulation tissue is formed. The presence of infection in the wound reduces the likelihood of "take" but it is not an absolute contraindication to grafting providing good drainage is achieved by, for example, the use of an expanded mesh graft or closed suction drainage under the graft. Presoaking the graft in a solution of aqueous penicillin and streptomycin prior to grafting of an infected wound has been advocated to improve graft survival.

(3) *Chronic granulating wounds.* FSGs can also be applied to some chronically granulating wounds. However, because the

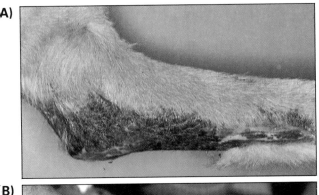

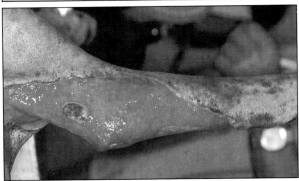

Fig. 5.2
(A) depicts a dog which suffered a large dermal abrasion following a road accident five days before. (B) the appearance of the same wound a few days later following surgical debridement and dressing until a suitable granulation tissue bed has formed.

superficial vascular supply is often poor in these cases it is important to remove surgically the top layer of tissue before grafting. If haemorrhage is extensive following this procedure it is advisable to bandage the wound for 24–48 h before grafting to avoid possible haematoma formation. Figure 5.3 shows a pale, poorly vascularized, chronic granulating wound and the appearance of the same wound after it has been surgically "freshened up".

HOW ARE FSGs HARVESTED?

The most suitable donor sites for skin in small animals are:

(1) The flank
(2) The lateral aspects of the cervical region

In these two sites there is normally plenty of mobile skin which can be removed while allowing the resulting deficits to be closed easily without creating undue tension. The FSG may be full or partial thickness.

(A)

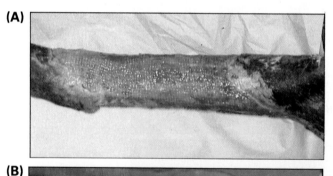

(B)

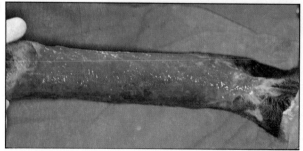

Fig. 5.3
(A) depicts a chronically granulating degloving injury in a dog following a road accident. (B) The appearance of the wound after removal of the superficial layer of the granulation tissue.

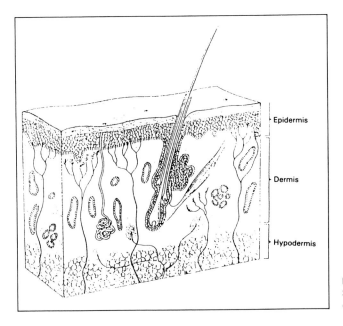

Fig. 5.4
Section through canine skin.

Full thickness grafts include epidermis and the whole of the dermis and are harvested by sharp dissection through the layer of loose connective tissue (the hypodermis) which separates the dermis from the underlying cutaneous trunci muscle (Figs 5.4 and 5.5). The resulting deficit can be closed

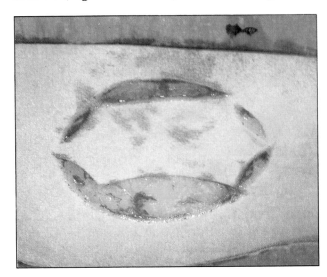

Fig. 5.5
A full thickness skin graft is being harvested from the flank leaving behind the underlying hypodermis.

by suturing first the subcutaneous and then the cutaneous tissues (Fig. 5.6).

Partial thickness grafts contain the epidermis with varying thicknesses of dermis. Harvesting this type of graft is more complex and is most easily performed using a dermatome, a rapidly oscillating mechanical blade, which ensures that an even thickness of skin is removed. Partial thickness grafts may be harvested by hand but it is often difficult to achieve a predictable and consistent depth of skin by this method. Donor sites are then left to heal without surgical closure and may often, therefore, develop an unsightly appearance. The advantages and disadvantages of full and partial thickness FSGs are summarized in Table 5.1.

Table 5.1 Advantages and disadvantages of full and partial thickness FSGs.

	Full thickness	Partial thickness
Cosmetic result	Good	Sparse hair cover, scarring at donor site
Durability	Good	More susceptible to trauma
Ease of harvesting	Simple	Ideally needs dermatome, hand harvesting is unsatisfactory
Ease of take	Poorer nutrition in early stages may result in some graft loss	Greater percentage take compared with full thickness
Availability of graft tissue	Limited to loose areas which can be reconstructed by primary repair	Greater proportion of skin available because primary repair not indicated, therefore useful for major skin defects, eg, burns

HOW ARE FSGs PREPARED AND APPLIED?

In order to promote initial adherence to the graft bed, as much of the underlying adipose and connective tissue should be removed from FSGs as possible. Partial thickness grafts however normally require little additional preparation. Both

A)

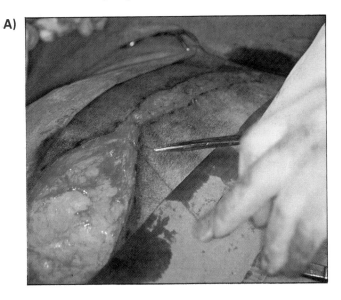

(B)

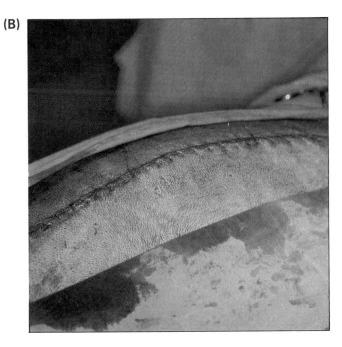

Fig. 5.6
(A) Closure of the subcutaneous tissue and (B) skin deficit created by the harvesting of a large FSG.

full or partial thickness grafts may then be used in a meshed or non-meshed form.

NON-MESHED GRAFTS

A template of sterile gauze is cut to fit accurately the shape of the recipient bed and the graft is harvested or modified to this shape. A few millimetres overlap at the wound edges is allowed for subsequent contraction of the graft.

MESHED GRAFTS

These are prepared by making rows of parallel incisions through the graft either by hand or with the help of a meshing instrument (Fig. 5.7). Once meshed the graft may be applied in varying degrees of expansion from minimal (Fig. 5.8) to fully expanded (Fig. 5.9).

The creation of a mesh has several advantages:

(1)   Improved drainage of fluids which accumulate below the graft

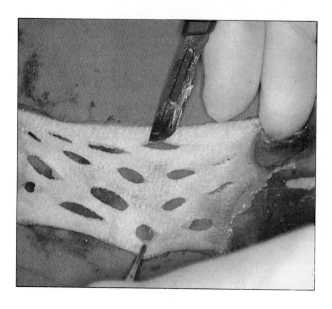

Fig. 5.7
Creation of parallel slits approximately 1 cm long and 1 cm apart using a scalpel to make a meshed FSG.

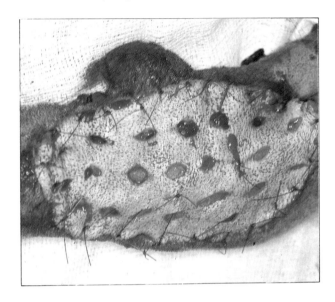

Fig. 5.8
Minimally expanded
FSG which has been
placed on the skin
wound seen in Fig.
5.1. Note placement
of sutures around the
edge of the graft and
through it to minimize
movement.

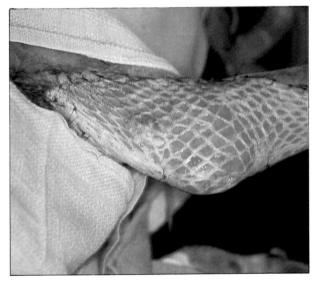

Fig. 5.9
Fully expanded mesh
graft (created using a
meshing instrument)
applied to the wound
seen in Fig. 5.3.

(2)   Greater conformation to uneven surfaces and irregular shaped wounds

(3)   Expansion to cover an area as much as two to three times the original width of the graft, although this will necessitate an additional lengthening of the graft when harvested.

Both full and partial thickness grafts should be orientated so that the direction of the hair growth matches that of the recipient area and then anchored with simple interrupted sutures of 3/0 monofilament nylon at their periphery. Care should be taken not to overtighten the sutures or to place too many in the graft which may interfere with revascularization. Where particularly large or uneven areas of skin are to be grafted it may be appropriate to use additional sutures through the graft surface to anchor it to the recipient bed below at various points.

HOW DOES AN FSG TAKE?

The process of graft "take" can be considered to have two components, graft adherence and graft nutrition.

GRAFT ADHERENCE

The initial adherence of the graft to the bed results from the development of fibrin strands between the FSG and the recipient area. This scaffolding of fibrin is then invaded by fibroblasts, leucocytes and phagocytes which strengthen the initial attachment by the production of collagen. This attachment increases in strength with time and is usually maximal by 10 days. The collagen produced in this site gradually matures and in so doing may cause contraction of the graft in the ensuing weeks. This is particularly noticeable in partial thickness grafts.

GRAFT NUTRITION

Nutrition by direct diffusion (plasmatic imbibition)

During the first 2–3 days the graft depends for its nutrition on absorption of a fibrinogen-free, serum-like fluid from the graft bed through its dermal capillaries and lymphatics. At this stage there is no circulation in the graft and it becomes engorged with this fluid taking on a bluish appearance.

Vascular nutrition

The ultimate viability of the graft depends on the development of an adequate arterial and venous supply between the graft and the graft bed. Approximately 1–2 days after grafting new vessels begin to develop from the graft bed, crossing the fibrin attachment and anastamosing with the dermal vessels of the graft (a process known as inosculation). Most of the long-term revascularization occurs, however, through the ingrowth of new vessels from the graft bed directly into the dermis of the graft or following the path of old dermal vessels. Revascularization is complete anytime between 4–12 days post grafting.

WHAT FACTORS WILL INTERFERE WITH THE TAKE OF FSGs?

As already indicated the long-term viability of the graft depends on the development of new blood vessels between the recipient bed and the graft. Anything which interferes with this process during the first week after grafting will therefore jeopardise the success of the graft.

PHYSICAL OR MECHANICAL SEPARATION OF THE GRAFT FROM THE BED

Accumulation of fluid below the graft

A seroma/haematoma will tend to separate it from the graft bed and impair the process of imbibition or hinder the development of revascularization. Haemostasis of the graft bed should therefore be thorough prior to graft placement. Where fluid accumulation can be expected (eg, grafting a recent wound or a very haemorrhagic granulation tissue), some provision for drainage should be made. This is most easily achieved by using a mesh graft but can also be achieved using closed suction drainage systems.

Movement of the graft over the bed

Graft immobilization during revascularization is important because any movement will disturb this process. Movement of the graft is prevented by:

(1) *Suturing.* The graft should not only be anchored at the periphery of the wound but also at strategic points through its surface to maintain contact with the graft bed.

(2) *Bandaging.* This is particularly important when grafting the extremities and a bandage incorporating a gutter splint should be used to aid immobilization. Attention to detail when bandaging is important and the following points should be considered:

(a) *Construction.* A non-adherent dressing is placed directly in contact with the graft to minimize disturbance of the graft when the dressing is changed. This may be either a non-adherent pad, eg, Melolin (Smith & Nephew) or if copious exudation is expected a petrolatum impregnated gauze dressing can be used. The intermediate layer of the dressing should be absorbent, eg, Velband (Johnson & Johnson), and combined with a conforming bandage. The outer layer should be strong, supporting and protective, eg, Vetrap (3M) or Elastoplast (Smith & Nephew). Fig. 5.10 illustrates a well-constructed bandage.

(b) *Frequency of change.* The graft should be disturbed as infrequently as possible during the first seven days *but* accumulation of exudate at the wound surface should be kept to a minimum. Thus the frequency of changing will

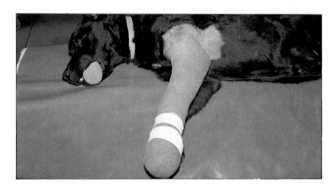

Fig. 5.10
A well-constructed bandage.

vary. In general, if a fresh wound is grafted copious exudate can be anticipated and the dressing may initially need to be changed daily. If, however, an established granulation tissue bed is grafted the dressing may be left in place for 3–4 days before a change.

(c) *Duration of bandaging*. This is a matter of judgement and experience but bandaging is usually maintained for 2–3 weeks until the graft has satisfactorily taken and, in the case of a mesh graft, re-epithelialization is complete.

Self mutilation

Steps should be taken to prevent the patient from mutilating the graft by means of adequate bandaging and, where necessary, Elizabethan collars.

SEPSIS

Infection interferes with graft take by causing cell death in both the graft and the bed. The initial fibrin attachment is dissolved and the migration of cells into the area is slowed, delaying revascularization. The area to be grafted should therefore be made as clean as possible prior to grafting. In infected wounds, topical rather than systemic antibiotics may be more effective, however care must be taken to choose an antibiotic preparation that will not hinder epithelialization. A combination of neomycin/polymixin/bacitracin in a spray preparation or silver sulphadiazine cream (Flamazine; Smith & Nephew) are recommended for this reason. Oily preparations such as intramammary drugs should *not* be used. In the presence of a heavily infected wound, systemic antibiosis may also be indicated. The antibiotic chosen should have activity against beta lactamase producing organisms.

WHAT HAPPENS TO AN FSG AFTER IT HAS TAKEN?

Once the graft has established its vascular supply epithelialization begins from the edges of each individual cell of the

mesh until the entire wound has re-epithelialized. This
sequence is illustrated in Fig. 5.11.

CONCLUSION

Free skin grafting is a simple technique which can be
undertaken with minimal equipment and is easily performed

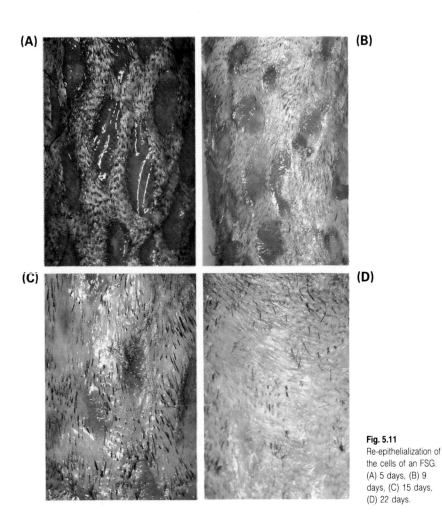

(A) **(B)** **(C)** **(D)**

Fig. 5.11
Re-epithelialization of
the cells of an FSG.
(A) 5 days, (B) 9
days, (C) 15 days,
(D) 22 days.

in general practice. With careful preparation and good post-operative care the technique can significantly reduce the healing time of a large cutaneous deficit and achieve an acceptable cosmetic result.

FURTHER READING

Probst, C. W., Peyton, L. C., Bingham, H. G. & Fox, S. M. (1983) *Journal of the American Animal Hospital Association* **19**, 555.

Swaim, S. F. (1980) *Management and Reconstruction in the Dog and Cat.* Philadelphia, W. B. Saunders.

Swaim, S. F. (1982) *Compendium of Continuing Education for the Practising Veterinarian* **4**, 194.

Swaim, S. F. (1985) *Textbook of Small Animal Surgery,* (ed. D. H. Slatter), p. 486. Philadelphia, W. B. Saunders.

Swaim, S. F., Pope, E. R., Lee, A. H. & McGuire, J. A. (1984) *Journal of the American Animal Hospital Association* **20**, 637.

Swaim, S. F., Lee, A. H., Newton, J. C. & McGuire, J. A. (1987) *Journal of the American Animal Hospital Association* **23**, 155.

CHAPTER 6

Fracture Fixation in Small Animal Practice

HAMISH DENNY

INTRODUCTION

Once a fracture has been reduced, and provided the blood supply to the fragments is intact, the main requirement for successful healing is the provision of adequate immobilization. The degree of stability achieved affects the size of callus formation; the more unstable the fracture the greater the size of the callus (Hutzschenreuter and others 1969). Conversely, a complete stable fracture should heal without callus formation. Rigid immobilization of a fracture can be achieved by internal fixation and compression of the fracture site. The aim of compression treatment of fractures is to achieve primary bone union in which direct longitudinal reconstruction of the bone occurs without any radiologically visible periosteal or endosteal callus (Muller and others 1970). Primary bone union should be striven for in the management of articular fractures but is not so essential in the management of diaphyseal fractures.

Is complete immobilization essential for healing? Fracture healing will proceed in the presence of a certain amount of tension, a considerable amount of bending will also be tolerated but torsion or rotation impedes healing because it causes tearing of the fibroblastic network of the callus and this may lead to non-union. Currently, the external fixator is the fashionable method of fracture fixation. The device can be used to vary the amount of movement at the fracture site, ie, rigid fixation during the early stages with an increase in micromovement or stress during the latter stages of healing. Studies have shown that controlled stress across the fracture both speeds the rate and improves the quality of bone healing (McKibbin 1978).

SELECTION OF APPROPRIATE METHOD OF FIXATION

DIAPHYSEAL FRACTURE

Fractures involving the diaphysics can be broadly divided into stable and unstable fractures.

Stable fractures are the transverse, blunt oblique or greenstick fractures in which the fragments interlock and resist shortening. The only fixation necessary is to prevent angular deformity and, depending on site, this may be done with either a cast, intramedullary pin, plate or external fixator.

The unstable fractures are oblique, spiral or comminuted. The fragments do not interlock. The method of fixation should maintain length of bone and prevent angulation and rotation. The ideal way of doing this is to reconstruct the bone with lag screws and apply a neutralization plate. If the fragments are too small for lag screw fixation, they are left *in situ* and a plate is applied to maintain bone length. In this situation, the plate acts as a buttress plate. The external fixator provides a useful alternative, is extremely versatile and can be used in the management of any diaphyseal fracture. It is the method of choice for fixation of open or infected fractures.

AVULSION FRACTURES

In an avulsion fracture, for example fracture of the tibial tuberosity, the fragment is distracted by the tensile force of the muscle tendon or ligament which inserts on the fragment. The fragment should be stabilized with Kirschner wires used in combination with a tension band wire to counteract the tensile force acting on the fragment.

ARTICULAR FRACTURES

In articular fractures, for example fracture of the lateral condyle of the humerus, early open reduction is essential to allow accurate reconstruction of the joint surfaces. Fixation is achieved with a transcondylar lag screw and a Kirschner wire to prevent rotation.

GROWTH PLATE FRACTURES AND SEPARATIONS

For growth plate fractures and separations early open reduction should be carried out. Kirschner wires are used for fixation (see below).

CLOSED REDUCTION AND CONSERVATIVE TREATMENT OF FRACTURES

Conservative methods of fracture treatment include:

(1) Cage rest
(2) Robert Jones bandage
(3) Thomas extension splint
(4) Casts and splints

CAGE REST

Pelvic fractures which involve non-weightbearing areas of the pelvis, ie, the pubis and the ischium, can be simply managed by confining the animal to a cage for 4–6 weeks. Cats with orthopaedic injuries seem to get better despite treatment, they respond well to cage rest and if there is doubt about the correct management of a pelvic or limb bone fracture in a cat then cage rest often gives satisfactory results.

ROBERT JONES BANDAGE, THOMAS EXTENSION SPLINT

These methods of fracture immobilization were described in Chapter 3. They tend to be used as a first-aid measure for temporary immobilization of fractures until internal fixation is carried out. The Robert Jones bandage is also often used for 5–10 days postoperatively to provide additional support and to control oedema.

CASTS AND SPLINTS

Casts or splints can be used as a definitive form of fracture treatment under the following criteria. The method should be reserved for stable fractures (greenstick, transverse, or blunt oblique). At least 50% of the fracture surfaces should be in contact following reduction for satisfactory healing to occur. It is desirable to immobilize the joint above and below the fracture, consequently the method is limited to fractures distal to the elbow and stifle. As a general rule, avulsion fractures and articular fractures should not be treated by closed reduction and external coaptation. Plaster of Paris is still a popular casting material but is tending to be superseded by fibreglass casting materials such as Vetcast (3M) and Zimflex (Zimmer) which are extremely strong and light.

MANAGEMENT OF FRACTURES IN GROWING ANIMALS

The management of fractures in puppies and kittens under five months of age differs from methods described for adult animals. The fractures heal very rapidly in 2–4 weeks. Plenty of callus is produced which undergoes rapid and complete remodelling, leaving little or no evidence of the original fracture. Closed reduction and external fixation should be used whenever possible in these immature animals. However, internal fixation has been recommended (Brinker and others 1983) when:

(1) The fracture results in excessive rotational deformity or shortening
(2) The fracture involves an articular surface and there is displacement
(3) The fracture involves a growth plate.

A small diameter intramedullary pin can be used for fixation of a shaft fracture because there is much more cancellous bone for the pin to embed in compared with the adult. Bone plates should rarely be used and are removed early (at approximately one month). Kirschner wires are used to reconstruct fractures involving joint surfaces, but in some cases a cancellous screw may be needed to give better stability.

The most important group of fractures affecting immature animals are those which involve the growth plate. Salter and Harris (1963) classified growth plate injuries into six types: Type 1 (epiphyseal separation) and Type 2 (separation of the epiphysis with fracture of a portion of the metaphysis) injuries are encountered most often. Reduction should be undertaken as early as possible—closed reduction and external fixation would be the ideal method of treatment but may be difficult to achieve owing to the small size of the epiphysis. In the majority of cases open reduction is necessary. This must be done with the minimum of trauma and care should be taken to avoid leverage on the epiphyseal side of the growth plate, otherwise the germinal cells will be damaged and premature closure caused.

If internal fixation is used, the ideal method is with Kirschner wires or small Steinmann pins placed across the growth plate with as little deviation from the long axis of the bone as possible (Fig. 6.1). Although this is the ideal placement, it is often easier to insert the Kirschner wires in a cruciate pattern (Fig. 6.2), and this should have little effect on longitudinal bone growth. The pins or Kirschner wires

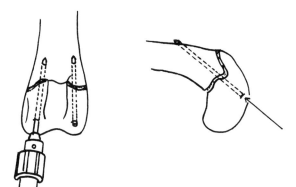

Fig. 6.1
Separation of the distal femoral epiphysis, fixation with parallel Kirschner wires.

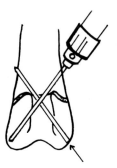

Fig. 6.2
Separation of the distal femoral epiphysis, fixation with crossed Kirschner wires.

should not occupy more than 20% of the surface area of the growth plate. Rush pins may also be used.

FRACTURE TREATMENT IN ADULT ANIMALS

INTRAMEDULLARY FIXATION

Intramedullary fixation is a simple method of fracture repair which is widely used in veterinary orthopaedics. The intramedullary devices include:

(1)   the Steinmann pin
(2)   the Rush pin
(3)   the Kirschner wire
(4)   the Kuntscher nail

The Steinmann pin is the most commonly used, the main indication being the treatment of stable fractures, ie, transverse or blunt oblique fractures of the middle third of long bones. As the pin lies within the medullary cavity it resists bending in all directions. Fracture stability is related to the tightness of the pin fit within the medullary cavity, interlocking of the fragments and muscle pull giving functional compression. The medullary cavity of long bones in the cat tends to be a uniform diameter so a tight pin fit can be achieved. In the dog, however, the medullary cavity varies in diameter so it is usually only possible to achieve three point fixation, one, at the point of insertion; two, at the fracture site or narrowest point of the medullary canal; and three by impacting the distal end of the pin into the cancellous bone of the metaphysis and epiphysis. A round intramedullary pin resists bending in all directions but has little resistance to shortening or rotation at the fracture site. Rotation or torsion is most likely to occur when a loose fitting pin is used for fixation and this may lead to non-union. Stability and resistance to rotation can be improved in several ways:

(1)   The intramedullary pin can be used in combination with an external fixator (Fig. 6.3)
(2)   In oblique fractures stability can be improved with cerclage or hemicerclage wiring
(3)   Instead of a single intramedullary pin, several narrower pins can be stacked within the medullary cavity
(4)   A Kuntscher nail which is V-shaped or clover leaf in cross section can be used instead of the intramedullary pin. This technique has largely been superseded by stacked pinning in small animal orthopaedics.

Although an intramedullary pin disturbs endosteal callus formation it causes little interference with the healing of the

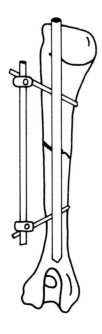

Fig. 6.3
Intramedullary pin used in combination with an external fixator for fixation of a humeral shaft fracture.

cortex and periosteum. Size of callus varies with stability achieved; if stability is good there will be minimal callus formation but if it is poor due to a loose fitting pin there will be extensive periosteal callus formation.

Intramedullary fixation should be avoided in comminuted fractures in dogs, the pin provides no longitudinal support or resistance to shortening forces and so collapse, rotation and non-union are to be expected. Cats are an exception; most shaft fractures in the cat, even if they are severely comminuted, can be successfully managed using a Steinmann pin in combination with cerclage wire (Figs 6.4 and 6.5). In the dog the intramedullary pin should be reserved for stable fractures of the middle third of the femoral or humeral shaft.

CERCLAGE WIRE

Cerclage wire is a wire loop that encircles the circumference of a bone. As indicated above, the wire is generally used in combination with an intramedullary pin to provide rotational

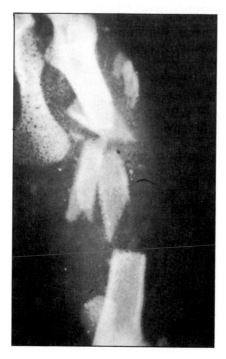

Fig. 6.4
Comminuted femoral shaft fracture in a two-year-old cat.

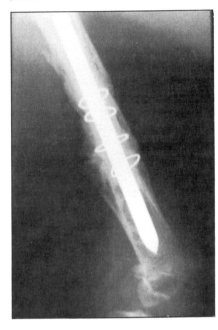

Fig. 6.5
Follow-up radiograph three months after fracture
repair with an intramedullary pin and multiple
cerclage wires. The fracture has healed.

stability in oblique or comminuted fractures. It is important
to apply cerclage wires correctly as a loose wire will cause
osteolysis and may lead to non-union. Guidelines for application of cerclage wire are listed below:

(1)   18 gauge (1.2 mm thickness) wire is used in animals over
20 kg in weight. In animals under 20 kg at least 20 gauge
(1 mm thickness) should be used.
(2)   The wire should be applied tightly and specific wire
tighteners are available for this purpose. The wire is tied
either by twisting or by the use of an ASIF loop (Fig. 6.6).

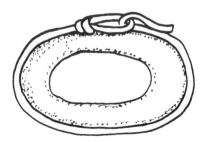

Fig. 6.6
The ASIF loop for tightening a cerclage wire.

(3)   In oblique fractures, the fracture line should be at least twice the length of the diameter of the shaft if shearing forces are to be resisted by the cerclage wire.
(4)   If multiple cerclage wires are used they should be spaced at least 1.0 cm apart.
(5)   To prevent the wire slipping either notch the bone or use a hemicerclage wire in which the wire penetrates the cortex of the bone via a drilled hole.

AO/ASIF principles of fracture repair

The AO group (The Association for the Study of Osteosynthesis) was formed by a group of Swiss surgeons in 1958. Later, the group became known as ASIF, the Association for the Study of Internal Fixation. The AO/ASIF group defined biomechanical principles for the successful treatment of fractures by internal fixation. The basic research was done at the Laboratory for Experimental Surgery in Davos, Switzerland. Metallurgical expertise was gained from the watch industry and an entire system of implants and instruments was developed for fracture treatment (Straumann; Straumann Great Britain; Veterinary Drug Company).

The aim of the AO/ASIF method is to restore full function to the injured limb as quickly as possible. This is achieved by:

(1)   Atraumatic surgical technique
(2)   Accurate anatomical reduction, especially in intra-articular fractures
(3)   Rigid internal fixation
(4)   The avoidance of soft tissue damage and fracture disease, ie, joint stiffness, muscle wasting and osteoporosis, by early mobilization.

Rigid fixation is achieved by compression techniques, which may take the form of:

(1)   Functional compression as in tension band wiring
(2)   Interfragmental compression which is achieved with lag screws

(3)   Axial compression, which is achieved with a plate or a wire using the tension band principle, in which the fixation device is placed on the tension side of the bone (Fig. 6.7).
(4)   Interfragmental compression used in combination with a neutralization plate or external fixator.

TENSION BAND WIRING

Tension band wiring is indicated for the treatment of avulsion fractures of the olecranon, greater trochanter, patella, tibial tuberosity, and os calcis. In all these fractures the fragment is distracted by the muscle, tendon or ligament which inserts on it. The tension band is placed so that it counteracts the tensile force acting on the fragment and redirects it to compress the fragment against the adjacent bone; this is functional compression and results from muscle pull (Pauwells 1965). The use of Kirschner wires and a tension band wire for the management of a tibial tuberosity avulsion is illustrated in Fig. 6.8.

INTERFRAGMENTAL COMPRESSION

Interfragmental compression is a method of compressing two fragments of bone together and is achieved by the lag screw principle. Any screw can be used as a lag screw, the lag effect is achieved by overdrilling the screw hole in the near fragment

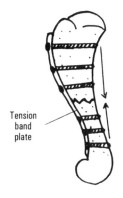

Tension band plate

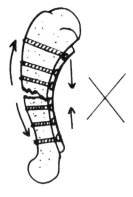

Fig. 6.7
Plates should be positioned on the tension side of bone. If applied to compression side, excessive bending results in plate fracture.

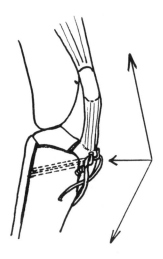

Fig. 6.8
Kirschner wires and a
tension band used for
fixation of an avulsion
fracture of the tibial
tuberosity. Arrows show
lines of force.

so that the screw thread grips in the far fragment only, then
when the screw is tightened the two bone fragments are
drawn together and the fracture line is compressed. Two types
of ASIF screws have been developed: the cortex screw for use
in the hard cortical bone of the diaphysis, and the cancellous
screw which has a coarser thread designed to achieve a better
purchase in the soft bone of the metaphysis and the epiphysis.
ASIF screws are not self-tapping, a tap is used to cut a thread
in the bone. This instrument removes bone debris and ensures
a good fit for the screw thread with minimal bone damage.
ASIF screws achieve a better purchase in bone compared with
the traditional self-tapping Sherman screws. Lag screw fixation
(usually in combination with a Kirschner wire to prevent
rotation) is used for the management of articular fractures
(Fig. 6.9).

Lag screws are also used in the reconstruction of oblique
or comminuted diaphyseal fractures, the repair is then
protected by the application of a neutralization plate (Fig.
6.10).

PLATE FIXATION

The use of a plate for fracture fixation should result in optimal
stability at the fracture site and allow early pain-free limb

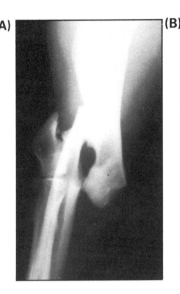
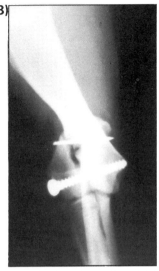

Fig. 6.9
(A) Preoperative radiograph of the elbow of a three-year-old springer spaniel showing fracture of the lateral humeral condyle. (B) Postoperative radiograph of the same dog; fixation has been achieved with a transcondylar lag screw and a Kirschner wire.

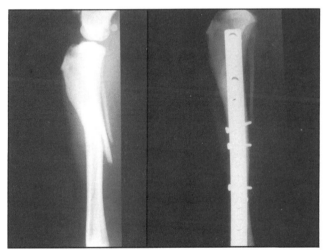

Fig. 6.10
(Left) Preoperative radiograph of a four-year-old boxer, showing an oblique mid shaft fracture of the tibia. (Right) Postoperative radiograph of the same dog showing reconstruction of the shaft using three lag screws to produce interfragmental compression followed by the application of a narrow 4.5 DCP as a neutralization plate on the medial aspect of the tibia.

function. The traditional Venables and Burns bone plates still have a useful place in the management of canine fractures particularly in medium-sized dogs. The Sherman and Lane plates are weak and their use is limited to small dogs and cats. The range of implant size is very limited when it comes to the management of fractures in giant breeds or miniature breeds of dog. The ASIF range of plates and screws provides the possibility of successful treatment of fractures in animals of any size (Fig. 6.11). ASIF plates are classified either by their type or function.

Plate type

Dynamic compression plate (DCP)

Figures below, eg, 4.5, apply to plate size and diameter of cortical screw used with plate.

(a)   4.5 DCP narrow or broad (used in large or giant breeds of dog)
(b)   3.5 mm narrow or broad (medium to large breeds of dog)
(c)   2.7 (small dogs or cats)
(d)   Mini DCP used with 2 mm cortex screws (toy and miniature breeds of dog, and cats).

Semitubular plate, (1/2, 1/3 or 1/4 segments)

The quarter tubular plate is the most useful, takes 2.7 mm screws, used in cats and small breeds of dog, also in mandibular fractures and acetabular fractures in dogs.

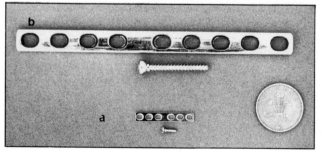

Fig. 6.11
AO/ASIF implants are made in a great range of sizes, demonstrated here are the mini DCP used with 2 mm cortex screws suitable for fixation in toy and miniature breeds and the narrow 4.5 DCP used with 4.5 mm screws in large and giant breeds of dog.

Small fragment plates

These come in a variety of shapes, "T" plates, angled plates, etc, used with 2.7 mm cortex screws, useful for pelvic fractures and mandibular fractures.

Mini plates

These can be used with 2 mm or 1.5 mm cortex screws. Useful for radius and ulna fractures in toy and miniature breeds of dog.

Special plates (Fig. 6.12)

(1) The reconstruction plate can be cut to length and contoured in any direction. It is especially useful in pelvic fractures.
(2) The acetabular plate is designed to curve around the dorsal acetabular rim.
(3) Double hook plates are designed to stabilize fractures and osteotomies near the ends of long bones.

There are other ASIF plates but the ones listed above are used most often in small animal orthopaedics.

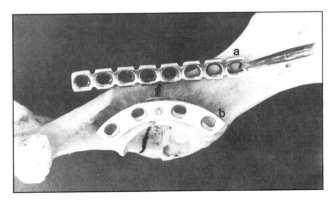

Fig. 6.12
Special AO/ASIF plates: (a) the reconstruction plate, this plate can be bent in any direction and cut if necessary, useful for pelvic fractures; (b) the curved acetabular plate designed to fit round the dorsal acetabular rim.

Plate function

Although DCP means dynamic compression plate the DCP is not always used as a compression plate, it may also function as a neutralization plate or as a buttress plate.

The dynamic compression plate (Allgower and others 1973)

The main feature of the DCP is the design of the screw hole which is based on the spherical gliding principle (Fig. 6.13). This enables the plate to be used as a self-compressing plate. Insertion of a screw in the load position will displace the bone beneath the plate towards the fracture site as the screw is tightened against the hemicylindrical slope of the screw hole. As the screws are tightened the plate is placed under tension and the fracture site is compressed. The loaded drill guide is generally used once on either side of the fracture. However, if further compression is needed, another screw may be inserted in the load position on either side of the

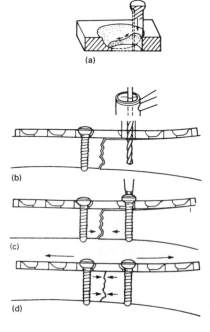

(a)

(b)

(c)

(d)

Fig. 6.13
Dynamic compression plate screw hole design.
(Redrawn with permission from Allgower.)

fracture. The remaining screws are placed using a neutral drill guide.

The greatest fracture gap that can be compressed is 3.2 mm with a 2.7 DCP, 4.0 mm with a 3.5 DCP and 4.0 mm with a 4.5 DCP.

The prime indication for compression plate fixation is a simple transverse diaphyseal fracture, eg, radius and ulna (Fig. 6.14). The method provides optimal stability at the fracture site and primary bone union should result.

The DCP can also be used to produce axial compression in oblique shaft fractures but in addition a lag screw is placed through the plate to produce interfragmental compression at the fracture site.

Neutralization plate

A neutralization plate is any plate which is used without compression. Typically a neutralization plate is applied after lag screws have been used to reconstruct the shaft in an

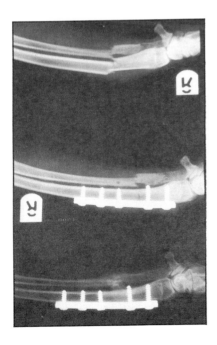

Fig. 6.14
(Top) Preoperative radiograph of a six-month-old Saluki showing transverse fracture of the distal third of the radius and ulna. Middle: Postoperative radiograph using a 4.5 DCP to compress the radial fracture site. (Bottom) Follow-up radiograph at six weeks. There is primary bone union at the radial fracture site. The only callus visible surrounds the ulnar fracture site which was not completely reduced.

oblique or comminuted fracture (Fig. 6.15). The plate is used to protect this repair and transmits all stresses from the proximal to the distal end of the bone.

Buttress plate

A plate which is used to span an area of comminution where the fragments are too small for lag screw fixation is called a buttress plate (Fig. 6.16).

EXTERNAL SKELETAL FIXATION

The external fixator is an extremely versatile method of fixation which can be used to stabilize a great variety of fractures and osteotomies. The Kirschner splint (Benkat) and the AO/ASIF external skeletal fixator (Straumann; Straumann GB) are used most often in small animal orthopaedics.

The external fixator is particularly suitable for open fractures with gross soft tissue damage, infected fractures or severely comminuted fractures (Fig. 6.17). The pins are placed at some distance away from the fracture site and are therefore less likely to encourage the spread of infection, the traumatized area is easily accessible for dressing, the device is relatively

(A)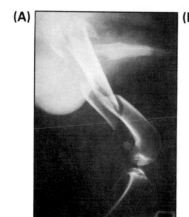
(B)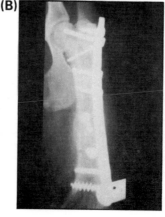

Fig. 6.15
(A) Preoperative radiograph of a five-year-old labrador. There are comminuted fractures involving the proximal and mid shaft regions of the femur. (B) Follow-up radiograph at four months showing that the fractures have healed. The shaft was reconstructed with lag screws and a 4.5 DCP was applied to the lateral side of the femur as a neutralization plate.

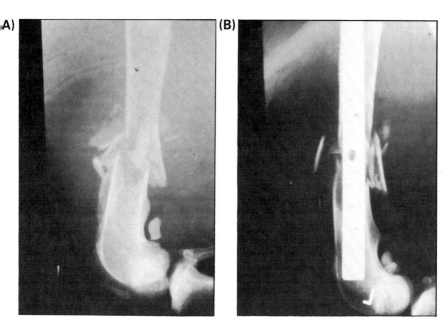

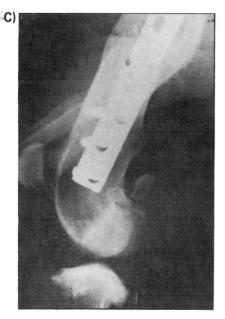

Fig. 6.16
(A) Preoperative radiograph of a five-year-old St Bernard, showing comminuted mid shaft frature of the femur. (B) Postoperative radiograph. A broad 4.5 DCP was applied as a buttress plate, the fragments were left *in situ*. (C) Follow-up radiograph at four months showing the fracture has healed.

H. Denny

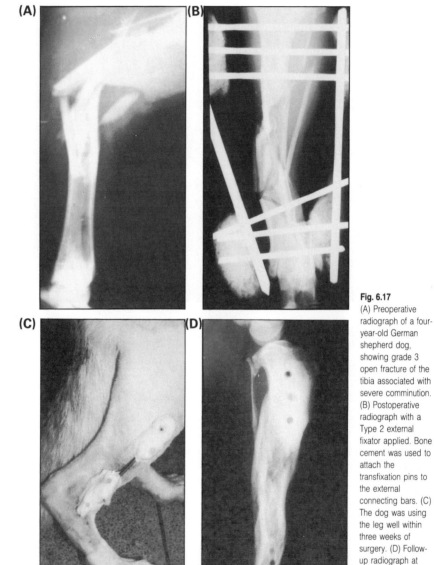

(A) **(B)** **(C)** **(D)**

Fig. 6.17
(A) Preoperative radiograph of a four-year-old German shepherd dog, showing grade 3 open fracture of the tibia associated with severe comminution. (B) Postoperative radiograph with a Type 2 external fixator applied. Bone cement was used to attach the transfixation pins to the external connecting bars. (C) The dog was using the leg well within three weeks of surgery. (D) Follow-up radiograph at three months. The fracture has healed and the external fixator was removed at this stage.

quick and easy to apply and the pins can be driven transcutaneously.

In its simplest form the method involves the transcutaneous insertion of two half pins each in the proximal and distal bone segments which are then connected to an external bar by clamps. If no clamps are available the external bar can be secured to the half pins with wire and cylinders of bone cement or technovit. The splint should be applied to the craniolateral surface of the humerus, craniomedial surface of the radius, lateral surface of the femur or medial surface of the tibia.

Various configurations of external fixator may be used which are beyond the scope of this paper, they can be unilateral (type 1), bilateral (type 2), or biplanar (type 3). For further information see Eggar (1983) and Brinker and others (1990).

FRACTURE HEALING TIME AND REMOVAL OF FIXATION DEVICES

Brinker (1978) defined clinical union as that time during the recovery when fracture healing had progressed sufficiently for the fixation device to be removed. He produced a table giving the average anticipated healing time for simple fractures in animals of different ages using different methods of fixation (Table 6.1).

Table 6.1 Time to reach clinical union (Brinker 1978).

Age of animal	External fixation External fixator Intramedullary pin	Plate fixation
Under 3 months	2–3 weeks	4 weeks
3–6 months	4–6 weeks	2–3 months
6–12 months	5–8 weeks	3–5 months
Over 1 year	7–12 weeks	5 months–1 year

112 *H. Denny*

REFERENCES

Allgower, M., Matter, P., Perren, S. M. & Reudi, T. (1973) *The Dynamic Compression Plate (DCP).* Berlin, Heidelberg, New York, Springer Verlag.
Brinker, W. O. (1978) *Small Animal Fractures.* East Lansing, Michigan, Department of Continuing Education Services, Michigan State University Press.
Brinker, W. O., Piermattei, D. L. & Flo, G. L. (1983) *Handbook of Small Animal Orthopaedics and Fracture Treatment,* p. 195. Philadelphia, W. B. Saunders Company.
Brinker, W. O., Piermattei, D. L. & Flo, G. L. (1990) *Handbook of Small Animal Orthopaedics and Fracture Treatment,* 2nd edn, pp. 24–28. Philadelphia, W. B. Saunders Company.
Egger, E. L. (1983) *Veterinary Surgery* **12**, 130.
Hutzschenreuter, P., Perren, P., Steinemann, S., Geret, V. & Klebl, M. (1969). *Injury* **1**, 77.
McKibbin, B. (1978) *Journal of Bone and Joint Surgery* **60B**, 150.
Muller, M. E., Allgower, M. & Willeneger, H. (1970) *Manual of Internal Fixation,* p. 19. Berlin, Heidelberg, New York, Springer Verlag.
Pauwells, F. (1965) *Gesammelte Aghandlungen zur Functionellen Anatomie les bewegungs-apparates.* Berlin, Heidelberg, New York, Springer Verlag.
Salter, R. B. & Harris, W. R. (1963) *Journal of Bone and Joint Surgery* **45A**, 587.

CHAPTER 7

External Support for Small Animals

COLIN STEAD

INTRODUCTION

External fixation is a method of fracture support where casts or splints are used until fracture healing takes place. External support is also used as a first aid measure for injured limbs and postoperatively. In the dog and cat, external support is chiefly used for injuries below the elbow or stifle joints and occasionally for neck and tail fractures.

FIRST AID AND POSTOPERATIVE SUPPORT

ROBERT JONES DRESSING

The Robert Jones dressing is commonly used as a postoperative support which helps to reduce oedema. It is an excellent first aid measure for lower limb fractures and may be applied over sterile dressings if wounds are present. It depends on the rigidity given by one or more rolls of cotton wool wrapped round the injured limb like a bandage. Halving the rolls of cotton wool first makes their application easier. The first stage in the dressing and indeed in that of almost any support is to attach long strips of adhesive tape (Elastoplast, zinc oxide, etc) down the front and back of the leg (Fig. 7.1). These strips should extend 10 cm beyond the tips of the toes. They serve to keep dressings and splints attached to the leg. Cotton wool is wrapped around the leg like a bandage until the required degree of splinting is obtained. The lengths of adhesive tape are then folded back up the leg front and back and the dressing is completed by incorporating them in a firm bandage applied in overlapping rolls, eg, Vetrap (3M) (Fig. 7.2). Despite its clumsy look this type of support is very comfortable and well tolerated by animals.

FINGER SPLINTS OR ZIMMER SPLINTS (Fig. 7.3)

These are foam-backed aluminium strips supplied in 46 cm lengths and in three widths from 12.5 to 25.5 mm (OEC Orthopaedic). They are useful as temporary supports but are not rigid enough for long-term use. They are easily bent to shape or cut to length and more than one may be used for extra rigidity. They should be contoured to the shape of the

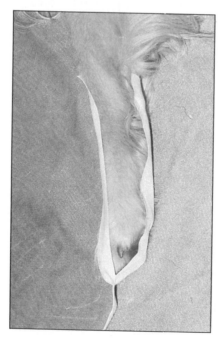

Fig. 7.1
Tape strips applied to the foot.

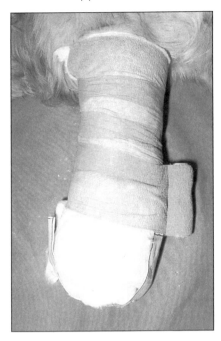

Fig. 7.2
Robert Jones dressing—tape strips folded up and being incorporated.

limb and bandaged in place over a padded dressing, normally to the front and back of the limb. To ensure the ends of the aluminium strip cannot dig into the soft tissues, they should be folded over.

A similar material is the Sam Splint produced in the USA (Seaberg & Associates). This is sheet aluminium sandwiched between two layers of foam plastic. It is much wider than the finger splints and malleable and can be used to construct gutter splints, cervical collars, etc. It is a potentially useful material.

GUTTER SPLINTS (Fig. 7.3)

Gutter splints are approximately $\frac{1}{3}$ to $\frac{1}{2}$ cylinder shaped lengths of plastic, metal or cast material. They may be purchased ready made in various sizes (Veterinary Drug) or constructed from cast material or plastic tubing. For forelimb use, a straight splint is satisfactory but for the hindlimb an angulation to allow a degree of hock flexion is desirable. The section of the splint should allow it to extend around three sides of the

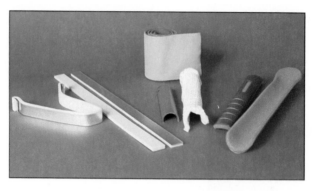

Fig. 7.3
Splints. Back, Sam splint.
Front left, Zimmer splints,
gutter splints of plastic,
Hexcelite, plastic
(Veterinary Drug).

bone to give maximum support. They are applied to the plantar or palmar surfaces of the limb after placing a double thickness of cast padding and are then bandaged firmly in place. Ensure that there are no sharp edges on the splint to cut into the soft tissues. They have the great advantage of easy removal and replacement for wound dressing.

FRACTURE REDUCTION

Reduction of a fracture requires general anaesthesia and good muscle relaxation. Suitable fractures for external fixation are transverse or short oblique fractures which are stable when reduced. If the fracture can be reduced but slips easily out of alignment, it is not suitable for external fixation. Fractures of the distal radius and ulna in animals over six months of age should be plated. Reduction depends on traction to reduce muscle spasm and angulation of the fracture tends to lever them together. Great care is necessary not to convert a closed fracture into a compound fracture by breaking the skin. If a fracture proves difficult to reduce, an open reduction and internal fixation should be carried out rather than causing extensive soft tissue damage. Occasionally a comminuted but undisplaced fracture of tibia with an intact fibula or one of radius or ulna with the other bone intact occurs. Such fractures are entirely suitable for external support.

UNDER-CAST PADDING (Fig. 7.4)

Many materials are available from different manufacturers. These range from cotton wool to synthetic bandage materials, stockinette and sheets of foam plastic. The rayon wool bandages (Soffban; Smith & Nephew, and Velband; Johnson & Johnson) are supplied in individual rolls and are very convenient to use and easier to apply than cotton wool which must be bandaged in place. They are also relatively cheap. Stockinette is also effective but the sheet foam materials are expensive.

Although under-cast padding is not always essential, it is more comfortable for the animal. Furthermore with some thermoplastic and resin casting materials the heat of the activation process is such that skin protection is required. The presence of under-cast padding is no guarantee that pressure sores will not occur. That depends on a stable, accurately contoured cast which has no ridges digging into the skin. Padding between the toes is unnecessary.

Before the padding is applied the anterior and posterior tape strips are placed and then an overlapping roll of padding applied from bottom to top so that there is a double thickness. It is a mistake to have too thick a layer, as this may allow undue cast movement and sores. The padding should extend above and below the proposed cast limits.

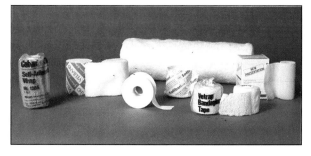

Fig. 7.4
Under-cast padding. Back, cotton wool. From left, Coban self-adhesive wrap (3M), Velband (Johnson & Johnson), zinc oxide tape (Paragon), Soffban (Smith & Nephew), Vetrap bandaging tape (3M), Elastoplast (Smith & Nephew).

GENERAL PRINCIPLES OF CAST APPLICATION

Casts are normally applied to limbs to approximate a standing position. However, when protecting a tendon repair, the limb is placed in such a way that the repaired tendon is relaxed. All casts, regardless of type, must include the whole foot or extend to the tips of the toes, leaving the two central pads exposed for weight bearing. It is dangerous to end a cast above the foot, as the circulation may be compromised distally (Fig. 7.5). A cast for a fracture of the radius and ulna need not extend above the elbow joint nor that for a fractured tibia above the stifle if they are properly applied, unless the fractures are very high on the bones.

After taping the foot and placing a double layer of cast padding, the cast itself is rolled on. Most cast materials are immersed in water for a few seconds, gently squeezed to remove surplus moisture and then applied firmly but not tightly in overlapping rolls taking care to contour the cast to the limb. Unnecessary ridges and depressions are avoided. Sufficient cast material is used to gain the required degree of rigidity and support. At some point the tape strips are folded up and included in the cast. Most casts will be hard to the touch in about three minutes. Particular care must be taken to roll out the top and bottom edges of the cast to avoid tissue pressure before rolling the cast padding down over the top edge and up over the bottom edge.

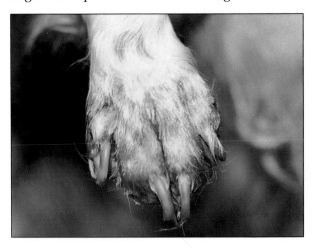

Fig. 7.5
Gangrenous foot caused by cast which stopped at distal metacarpus (note depression where cast stopped).

With plaster casts the slab technique may be used where longitudinal strips of plaster bandage two to four layers thick and the length of the proposed cast are smoothed into place to form a shell around the limb. Once hardened, further plaster bandage is applied in overlapping rolls to finish. This method obviates any risk of ischaemia from too tight a cast or shrinkage in drying.

Gutter splints may be constructed by making a complete cast shell and splitting it longitudinally with a plaster saw and discarding the anterior portion. One may also use the two half shells taped together as an easily removable cast where there are underlying wounds which need dressing. For the hind leg a below the knee cast has been described (Nunamaker 1985) which is in effect a half shell of cast applied to the dorsum of the limb from the stifle down and bandaged into place.

CASTING MATERIALS (Fig. 7.6)

There are three basic materials in common use for casts.

(1) Plaster of Paris and its modifications
(2) Thermoplastic materials
(3) Resin impregnated bandages

A selection of some of the commonly available materials is described and compared in Tables 7.1 and 7.2. The list is not exhaustive.

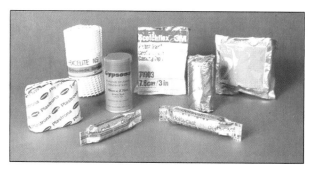

Fig. 7.6
Casting materials. From left, Plastrona (Hartmann), Hexcelite (Alfred Cox), Gypsona (Smith & Nephew), Scotchflex (3M), Cellamin (Lohmann), Scotchcast Plus (3M). Front, Delta Cast (Johnson & Johnson).

Table 7.1 Comparison of some casting materials and their application.

Product	Manufacturer/agent	Material	Gloves	Application			Ease of application*
				Water temp. (°C)	Immersion time	Time to harden (min)	
Gypsona	Smith & Nephew	Plaster of Paris	No	25–30	3.5 s	3	++
Plastrona	Hartmann	Plaster of Paris	No	20	3.5 s	3	++
Cellamin	Lohmann	Plaster of Paris and resin	Yes	20	2 s	3	++++
Hexcelite	Alfred Cox	Thermoplastic polymer	Yes (rubber)	70	5–60 min	3	+
Delta Cast	Johnson & Johnson	Polyurethane resin	Yes	20	3 s	5	+++
Scotchflex	3M	Fibreglass tape	Yes	20	3 s	3	++ (without hand cream)
Scotchcast Plus	3M	Fibreglass tape	Yes	20	3 s	2	++++

*Best ++++ (subjective opinion)

Table 7.2 Comparison of some casting materials and their application.

Product	Water resistance	Porosity*	Radiolucency*	Casting of standard fracture in a dog			Cast cost (£)	Removal
				Cast weight immediate (g)	Dry weight (g) and Time (h)	Number of rolls		
Gypsona	No	+	+	310	240 (120)	2 (10 cm)	0.72	Shears
Plastrona	No	+	+	340	260 (120)	2 (3 inches)	1.98	Shears
Cellamin	Yes	+	+	250	230 (72)	2 (10 cm)	0.80	Shears
Hexcelite	Yes	+ + + +	+	110	110 (<1)	1 (3 inches)	0.80	Shears/saw
Delta Cast	Yes	+ + +	+ + + +	100	100 (<1)	2 (10 cm)	4.58	Shears
Scotchflex	Yes	+ + +	+ +	75	75 (<1)	1 (3 inches)	6.33	Shears
Scotchcast Plus	Yes	+ +	+	160	160 (<1)	1 (3 inches)	8.11	Saw

*Best + + + + (subjective opinion)

Gloves Gloves are recommended when applying most casting materials to protect the operator's hands from chemicals and, in the case of Hexcelite, from the heat of the activation process. Vinyl or rubber gloves may be employed (eg, used operating gloves) except with Hexcelite, to which vinyl gloves stick.

Temperature All the agents are activated by water immersion and for Hexcelite the activation temperature of 70°C is critical. Manufacturer's recommended temperatures should be followed (basically tepid tap water). Increased temperatures speed up setting times and vice versa, but setting of Hexcelite may be speeded by dousing the cast in cold water (Edwards and Clayton Jones 1978). Two to five seconds of immersion suffice for all agents except Hexcelite, which requires a minimum of five minutes. When squeezing out wet bandages, standard plaster loss materials like Gypsona leave a lot of plaster in the bowl, whereas low plaster loss materials like Plastrona leave very little. There is no loss with resin or thermoplastics.

Application Ease of application of the materials varies. Plasters are messy to handle and a practised touch is needed to produce a smooth, even finish. Cellamin is outstandingly easy to apply and mould. Hexcelite is very difficult to apply and mould if the activation temperature is too low, but a dry cast can be modified by using hot air from a hairdryer or hot air gun to soften it. Scotchflex will stick to gloves unless the manufacturer's hand cream is used. Scotchcast Plus is very easy to apply and mould. All materials give off some heat as they dry, particularly Scotchcast Plus. The curing and lamination of Delta Cast is aided by applying a firm wet bandage to the cast as it dries. The speed of the initial hardening process means that all casts, regardless of type, have to be contoured smartly to their final form. Although all the materials feel hard within a few minutes and can reasonably be expected to stand weightbearing on recovery from anaesthesia, the plaster materials can take up to five days to dry and achieve their maximum strength. The resin casts and Hexcelite are much stronger than plasters (Houlton and Brearley 1985). Plaster of Paris casts are not water resistant and will soften if they become wet. They also allow little circulation of air. The resin and thermoplastic agents are water resistant and porous and the open weave of Hexcelite is outstanding in this respect.

Radiography The value of radiography through a cast varies. With the exception of Delta Cast, which is remarkably radiolucent, all the cast materials which I compared made radiographic interpretation through the cast difficult (Figs 7.7 and 7.8). Assessment of fracture reduction is usually possible but assessing fracture healing is more problematic. In general, a wet plaster cast needs a doubled exposure while a dry cast needs an increase of half. Other cast agents should require no adjustment of exposure factors.

Drying I compared the various materials in supporting a fractured radius and ulna in a 15 kg cadaver dog. Casts were applied over a double layer of Velband using 7.5 to 10 cm rolls of the cast materials. After initial hardening, the limbs were radiographed, the casts were removed and weighed and the weighing repeated at 24 hour intervals for five days to

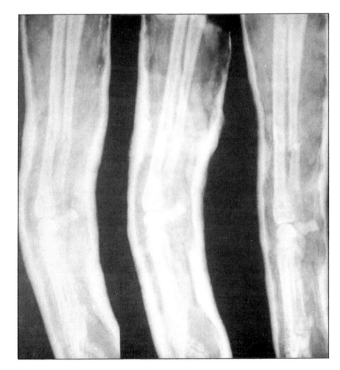

Fig. 7.7
Radiography through
a cast at 57 kV
5mAs. From left,
Gypsona, Plastrona,
Cellamin.

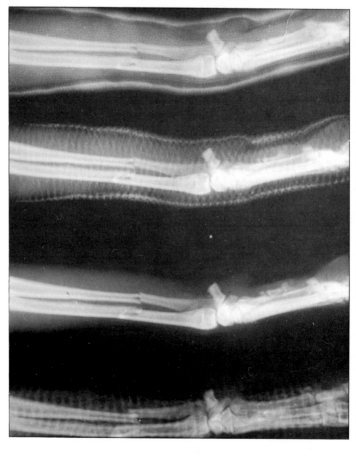

Fig. 7.8 Radiography through a cast at 57 kV 5mAs. From left, Hexcelite, Delta Cast, Scotchflex, Scotchcast Plus.

assess drying. The plaster casts took 96 to 120 hours to dry fully at room temperature as indicated by the final weight achieved. The thermoplastic and resin materials showed no weight change after their initial removal. They were also substantially lighter than the plaster agents. The roll lengths were fairly similar and two rolls were necessary to complete each cast except with Hexcelite and Scotchcast Plus which only needed one roll of each. Although only one roll of Scotchflex was used the cast felt marginally flimsy. The cost of each cast is based on NHS prices and gives an approximate price comparison. This does not include any addition for disposable gloves.

Removal The casts were compared for ease of removal. Plaster shears were satisfactory for all the materials except Scotchcast Plus for which an electric plaster saw was necessary although all the non-plaster material casts were harder to remove.

Softening All the casts were immersed in a bucket of cold water at room temperature for 24 hours and then examined for changes. Gypsona and Plastrona softened in that time, but the other casts including Cellamin appeared unaffected.

With casting materials, the advantages of greater strength, lighter weight and water resistance are expensive. Plaster of Paris as typified by Gypsona, for all its disadvantages, is both cheap and effective although Cellamin has significant advantages at not much greater cost. The resin agents have good "handleability", outstanding in the case of Scotchcast Plus. These and Hexcelite are strong, dry quickly and are water resistant. Delta Cast's remarkable radiolucency makes X-ray monitoring easy. An additional advantage of these materials is that their hardness makes patient interference more difficult but not impossible. Their main disadvantage is their greatly increased cost, against which fewer cast changes may be needed.

CAST REMOVAL

Cast removal is a tedious business and may require sedation of the animal. Plaster shears, old bone cutting forceps and plaster saws, hand or electric may be used (Fig. 7.9). Electric plaster saws are very quick and convenient and will not

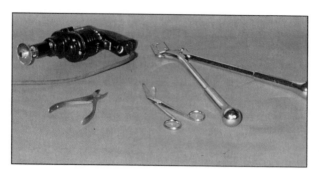

Fig. 7.9
Cast removal tools. From left, oscillating saw, old bone cutting forceps, dressing scissors, plaster shears.

damage soft tissues, but animals hate their noise and vibration and good restraint is essential.

THOMAS SPLINTS (Fig. 7.10)

These are extension splints custom made for each animal. They may be used for treatment or temporary support of

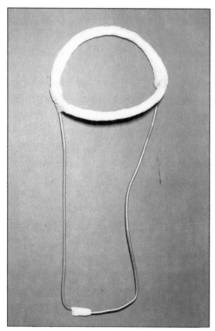

Fig. 7.10
Thomas splint for hind leg.

lower limb fractures. Their correct application requires great skill and they are now unpopular. They are made from aluminium rods of 2–4 mm diameter and 2 m length. A rod is bent round a wooden former to make a ring of sufficient size to encircle the animal's thigh or axilla. The ring is angled some 45° from its mid point and is then padded and taped to fit the inguinal or axillary area. The anterior bar is shaped to the standing leg. The lower ends of the bars are bent at right angles to form a walking bar to which the toes are taped with zinc oxide tape. The hock is bandaged to the posterior bar and the upper tibia is bandaged to the anterior bar to apply traction to the fractured bone for a tibial or distal femoral fracture. In the fore leg the elbow area is strapped to the posterior bar and the carpus to the anterior bar. Care is required to ensure that the limbs are not rotated in the splint or a malunion may result.

POSTOPERATIVE CARE

As a minimum, the veterinary surgeon must check any cast or splint weekly. Owners require clear instructions that in the event of their pet chewing a cast, the presence of a smell from the cast or signs that the animal is uncomfortable, increasingly lame or unwell, then they must return the animal promptly for veterinary examination. Interference with a cast or splint by the patient is a common problem and the only effective deterrent is the Elizabethan collar or similar device.

Casts will require changing in the course of treatment if they have been applied over a swollen leg, as the cast will reduce swelling and then loosen. For this reason, it is often better to reduce swelling by using a Robert Jones dressing first before casting. A cast will also loosen with muscle atrophy. A loose cast gives poor support and will cause sores.

Typically a fracture will need support for about six weeks, but sometimes longer and, before discarding all support, clinical and radiographic assessment of the fracture healing should be made to ensure that there is both stability and evidence of a mineralized bridging callus.

CAST COMPLICATIONS

The most common problem is that of pressure sores resulting from poor cast contouring and looseness. Wound dressing and recasting is then necessary. Ending a cast above the end of the foot or patient interference so that the bottom of the cast is chewed back to leave an edge which cuts into the dorsum of the foot leads to swelling and ischaemia distally. Should this be neglected, gangrene ensues with inevitable loss of limb.

Malunion of a fracture may occur caused by poor alignment of the fracture initially or by discarding support too early before a mineralized bridging callus is established. Non-union is a serious problem which results normally from inadequate reduction of the fracture or instability. The distal radius and ulna is an area notorious for non-union, especially in toy dogs. Delayed union is a fracture in which repair is slower than normal. It should be differentiated from a non-union and provided support is maintained will eventually heal.

AVIAN FRACTURES

Avian fractures heal faster than in mammalian bone, typically in about three weeks under good conditions.

LIMBS

(1) Fractures from distal femur downwards can be suitable for external support.
(2) Identification rings or jesses may need to be removed.
(3) Cast materials can be used as in small animals but patient interference can be a problem and the resin materials with their harder finish are more beak-resistant. Elizabethan collars can be made from stout cardboard.
(4) Useable splints can be made from lengths of malleable plastic tubing split longitudinally, slipped over the suitably padded limb and taped in place. With very small birds, splints may be made from zinc oxide tape and matchsticks.

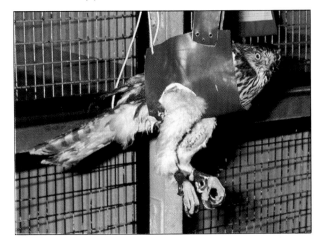

Fig. 7.11
Leather sling to support
goshawk with bilateral
limb fractures.

(5)   A bird with both limbs fractured may be supported initially in a leather body sling suspended from a hook (Fig. 7.11). In such a case the wings must be taped to the body to prevent struggling.

WINGS

(1)   As a first aid measure and to supplement external fixation, a fractured wing may be taped to the tail with zinc oxide tape to prevent it drooping and suffering further damage. For greater immobilization, the wing may be taped to the body (Fig. 7.12).

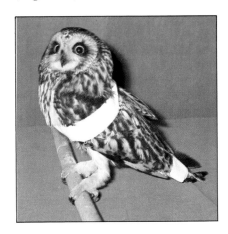

Fig. 7.12
A short-eared owl with fractured humerus. The
injured wing is taped to body and tail for temporary
immobilization of the fracture.

(2)   The full length of an avian wing is accessible for external support but most humeral fractures are oblique spiral in nature and unsuited to external support alone.

(3)   Fractures of the radius or ulna alone need minimal support as the intact bone splints the other. Suitable radius and ulna or metacarpal fractures may be supported with gutter-type splints applied to the leading edge of the wing along the line of the fractured bone. These splints, can be made from sheet aluminium, Sam splint or cast material taped into position. Coles (1985) has described the use of Hexcelite or X-ray film similarly applied but anchored behind the ulna with sutures passed through the splint into the skin and between the secondary feather shafts.

REFERENCES

Coles, B. H. (1985) *Avian Medicine and Surgery*. Oxford, Blackwell Scientific Publications.

Edwards, G. B. & Clayton Jones, D. G. (1978) *Veterinary Record* **102**, 397.

Houlton, J. E. F. & Brearley, M. J. (1985) *Veterinary Record* **117**, 55.

Nunamaker, D. M. (1985) *Textbook of Small Animal Orthopaedics* (eds C. D. Newton and D. M. Nunamaker). Philadelphia, J. B. Lippincott Co.

CHAPTER 8

Non-manual Restraint of Small Animals for X-ray

FRANCES BARR and JEANNE LATHAM

INTRODUCTION

The introduction of the Ionising Radiation Regulations 1985 and the associated Code of Practice has made it necessary to take a closer look at the way that radiography procedures are carried out in veterinary practice. The Code of Practice states that "only in exceptional circumstances should a patient or animal undergoing a diagnostic examination be supported or manipulated by hand". The veterinary surgeon is now obliged by law to follow this recommendation. This article suggests some ways in which non-manual restraint of small animals can be employed without compromising radiographic technique or endangering the patient.

There are certain radiographic examinations which, in the view of the authors, are best carried out under general anaesthesia as accurate positioning is critical. Such examinations include most views of the skull and pharynx, radiographs of the cervical, thoracic and lumbar spine, and radiographs of the pelvis which are to be submitted for evaluation under the BVA/KC hip dysplasia scheme.

Conversely, there are certain radiographic examinations for which general anaesthesia is contraindicated—notably barium studies of the oesophagus, stomach and small intestine.

With these exceptions, the choice of whether or not to use general anaesthesia rests with the clinician and will depend on many factors including the clinical condition and temperament of the animal. However, it is possible to carry out many radiographic examinations with the animal conscious if the techniques described below are employed in conjunction with judicious use of sedatives and tranquillizers.

CORRECT POSITIONING

The aim is to position the animal correctly according to basic radiographic principles, while achieving adequate restraint. The comfort of the patient must always be considered as an uncomfortable animal will rarely lie still. As soon as the animal is settled, personnel may leave the immediate vicinity of the X-ray table and an exposure be made.

Items we have found useful for positioning and restraint include (see Table 8.1):

(1) Moderately heavy floppy sandbags which may be draped across the patient or wrapped around limbs to simulate manual restraint. They should be long and thin, and only loosely filled. Cloth inner bags covered with proofed nylon are easy to clean and are virtually waterproof.

Table 8.1 Positioning aids and suggested sizes.

Positioning aids	Suggested sizes
Floppy sandbags	45 cm × 10 cm – 1.5 kg 60 cm × 12.5 cm – 2.4 kg 60 cm × 15 cm – 3 kg
Foam troughs	30 cm long × 15 cm wide × 10 cm high 45 cm long × 18 cm wide × 20 cm high 45 cm long × 30 cm wide × 20 cm high 45 cm long × 35 cm wide × 30 cm high
Foam wedges Polystyrene blocks Bandages/tapes Plastic reels Commercial positioning aids	

(2)   A selection of radiolucent foam troughs in which animals can be positioned comfortably in dorsal or ventral recumbency. These can be made from foam pieces stuck together with contact adhesive and covered with proofed nylon. It is important that the sides are thick enough to remain vertical when the animal is placed in them. Thin sides bow outwards and provide reduced restraint.
(3)   A selection of radiolucent foam wedges and shapes, which may be made or purchased from any of the suppliers of X-ray accessories. Polystyrene blocks can also be useful.
(4)   Cotton bandages or tapes for limb positioning. Sticky tape or Elastoplast can be employed to restrain very small animals or birds, although Elastoplast is not completely radiolucent at low exposures.
(5)   The plastic centres from reels of Elastoplast, which make convenient radiolucent gags and are particularly useful for dental radiography.

LATERAL THORAX POSITIONING (Fig. 8.1)

The animal is placed in lateral recumbency with one or more sandbags draped over the neck. The front legs must be drawn well forward and held in place with a sandbag wound around each carpus. One or more sandbags are similarly used to restrain the hind legs. It is often useful to drape a sandbag across the back and abdomen just in front of the pelvis. Finally, a foam wedge is placed under the sternum to achieve a true lateral position.

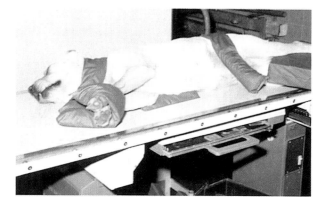

Fig. 8.1
Lateral thorax
positioning.

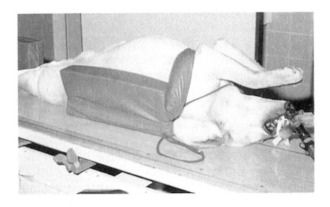

Fig. 8.2
Ventrodorsal pelvis
positioning.

VENTRODORSAL PELVIS POSITIONING (Figs 8.2
and 8.3)

The animal is placed in dorsel recumbency in a foam trough.
Twisting or rotation of any part of the body makes it difficult
to achieve perfect pelvic positioning, so sandbags and wedges
are used as necessary to position the thorax and front legs
symmetrically. The hind legs must be fully extended so that
the femurs are parallel to each other and to the cassette. A

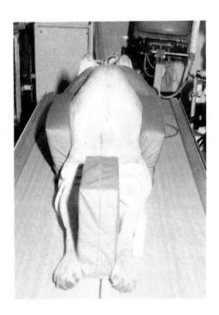

Fig. 8.3
Ventrodorsal pelvis positioning.

pad is placed between the hocks or stifles and a tape is tied firmly around both legs at the level of the mid thigh. If necessary a heavy sandbag is draped over each stifle to keep the legs down close to the table. Final fine adjustment can then be made to eradicate any pelvic tilt before leaving the immediate vicinity of the X-ray table and taking the radiograph.

DORSOVENTRAL THORAX POSITIONING (Fig. 8.4)

The animal is placed in sternal recumbency, with the front and hind legs positioned symmetrically on each side of the trunk to avoid rotation or twisting. A sandbag across the lumbar spine keeps the hindquarters down. The head and neck should be extended forwards and held down by a sandbag to avoid superimposition of the neck muscles on the cranial lung fields.

Similar principles can be applied to achieve accurate positioning of any part of the body without resort to manual

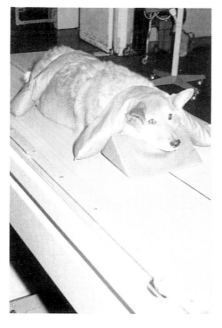

Fig. 8.4
Dorsoventral thorax positioning.

restraint other than in very exceptional clinical circumstances. This allows the veterinary surgeon to comply with the Ionising Radiation Regulations 1985 and the Code of Practice without compromising the condition of the animal or radiographic principles.

Additional positioning aids are commercially available, details of which may be obtained from suppliers of X-ray accessories.

Precisely which aids are used is largely a matter of personal preference and is not important provided the animals are positioned accurately and restrained comfortably without manual support.

FURTHER READING

Webbon, P. M. (1981) *A Guide to Diagnostic Radiography in Small Animal Practice*. Cheltenham, BSAVA Publications.

CHAPTER 9

Chemical Restraint for Radiography in Dogs and Cats

POLLY TAYLOR

INTRODUCTION

Chemical restraint for radiography is required to produce an animal that is quiet, malleable and preferably pain-free. Sedation must be sufficient to allow the animal to be restrained in position with sandbags and cradles so that all except the patient remain behind protective screens during exposure. Immediately after the relatively short procedure central nervous system (CNS) and cardiopulmonary depression must be minimal so that the animal is safe to leave, and, ideally, is able to walk.

There is a wide range of sedative and analgesic drugs suitable for use in the dog and cat, and it is usually feasible to adjust the dose of drug to achieve a predictable degree of sedation. Some sedative drugs are sufficient when used on their own, but it is often more satisfactory to use synergistic combinations of a sedative with an opiate analgesic. Some short-acting intravenous anaesthetic agents can also be used for the same purpose.

SEDATIVES: USE WITH CARE (Tables 9.1–9.4)

All sedatives, opioid analgesics and anaesthetics depress the CNS, and respiratory and cardiovascular depression are usually the most serious side effects. Excessive depression of these two systems must always be regarded as a potential hazard of chemical restraint.

Table 9.1 Drugs available for sedation.

Acepromazine

Widely used, mild sedative, usually insufficient on its own for radiography

Increasing the dose does not increase the sedation, only the side effects (long duration, hypotension)

May "release inhibitions" in some animals so they become unmanageable

Very useful in combination

Xylazine

Potent sedative with a deep and predictable response

Severe cardiovascular and respiratory depressant

If general anaesthesia is required later, induction and maintenance dose of all agents must be reduced by at least one half

Vomiting, which appears particularly distressing to the animal, should not be used as a routine method to ensure an empty stomach

Combinations with other sedatives or opiates are not recommended as they are likely to have a very depressant effect

Medetomicline is a close relative to xylazine which is new to the market. Its effects are similar to xylazine in many ways

Diazepam

Mild tranquillizer which, on its own, may induce bizarre behaviour

Little cardiovascular or respiratory depression

Chemically incompatible with other drugs—do not mix in the syringe

Injection, especially intramuscular (im), is painful (lipid formulation available for intravenous (iv) injection is less painful)

Useful in combination

Midazolam is water-soluble relative of diazepam which is shorter acting, less painful on injection, can mix with some other drugs in syringe (eg, opioids) but is otherwise similar to diazepam

Table 9.2 Opioids.

Morphine, methadone, pethidine, papaveretum, fentanyl, etorphine

These are pure agonists, are reversible with naloxone, and are controlled drugs (schedule 2 in Medicines Act 1968)

Buprenorphine, pentazocine, butorphanol

These are mixed agonist antagonists, need high doses of naloxone for reversal and are POM only (pentazocine control more stringent, schedule 3)

All opioids

Produce little sedation on their own (except etorphine which is very potent)

Most are respiratory depressant (etorphine and fentanyl especially)

Very good analgesia

Some may induce vomiting (morphine, papaveretum)

Little cardiovascular depression (except etorphine, causes hypotension in dogs)

Cats may exhibit bizarre excitement with morphine if given a slight overdose—etorphine and fentanyl are not recommended in cats

Synergism with sedatives, very useful for combinations

Table 9.3 Sedative agent dose rates.

Drug	Dose on own (mg/kg)	Comment
Acepromazine	0.02–0.1 im	Mild sedation. Reduce dose in large breeds
Xylazine	1–3 im	Profound sedation. Vomiting
Diazepam	up to 10 iv	Little sedation. May induce bizarre behaviour

Pre-operative examination is just as important before sedation as before general anaesthesia. A pre-existing condition that is not immediately life threatening in the conscious animal may become fatal under mild CNS depression and abnormal positioning. For instance, an animal with a thoracic mass may show few overt signs when sitting or standing, fully conscious. However, if its normal reflexes and cardiopul-

Table 9.4 Opioid dose rates.

Drug	Dose on own (mg/kg)	Comment
Buprenorphine	0.01	The opiates produce little
Methadone	0.1–0.2 CD	sedation on their own but
Morphine	0.2 (cat 0.1) CD	potentiate the effect of
Pentazocine	2	sedatives and general
Pethidine	2 CD	anaesthetics
Papaveretum	0.4 (not cats) CD	

CD Controlled drug Schedule 2

Table 9.5 Drug combinations.

Combinations of morphine, papaveretum, methadone, pethidine, pentazocine or buprenorphine with acepromazine are all effective in the dog. It usually results in a quiet and pliable animal that can stand and walk if encouraged.

Buprenorphine with acepromazine is now probably the preferred combination for radiography and has been used in thousands of dogs.

Acepromazine with pethidine, buprenorphine or pentazocine can be used in the cat.

Combinations of diazepam or midazolam with opioids are useful in old or debilitated animals (they cause less cardiovascular depression), however, it usually provides insufficient sedation in young healthy individuals.

Etorphine is marketed with the phenothiazine methotrimeprazine (Small Animal Immobilon; C-Vet).

Fentanyl is marketed with the haloperidol fluanisone (Hypnorm; Janssen).

Immobilon and Hypnorm are not suitable for cats and best avoided in debilitated dogs.

Immobilon and Hypnorm induce deeper sedation and respiratory depression than combinations with buprenorphine, morphine, etc, dogs appear virtually anaesthesized, but relaxation is variable.

Immobilon (etorphine component) is reversed with diprenorphine (Revivon; C-Vet) which results in return to near normal consciousness.

Hypnorm is usually not reversed, sedation may last over an hour.

monary function are depressed and it is positioned on its
back for radiography there will be drastic reduction in
functional lung which is likely to be rapidly fatal. Chest injury
or disease is the major case where it may be necessary for
the animal to be restrained manually; such an animal must
be allowed to adopt a position that it finds comfortable, and
should never be turned on its back.

It is all too easy to forget to monitor the animal that is
"only sedated", since it appears less depressed than if under

Table 9.6 Drug combination dose rates.

Drug	Dose	Comment
Dog		
Acepromazine ⎫	0.03–0.08 mg/kg*	im Onset approx 5–10 min. No
Buprenorphine ⎭	4–13 μg/kg	particular advantage from iv
Can substitute buprenorphine with		
papaveretum	20 mg	Total dose in large (40–50 kg) dog
or		
Pentazocine	1–2 mg/kg	
or		
Methadone	0.1–0.2 mg/kg	
or		
Pethidine	1–2 mg/kg	
Diazepam ⎫	up to 10 mg total dose	iv Better than acepromazine combinations in debilitated
Methadone ⎭	0.1–0.2 mg/kg	dogs Do not mix in syringe
Cat		
Acepromazine ⎫	0.05–0.2 mg/kg	im
Pethidine ⎬	2–4 mg/kg	
Atropine ⎭	0.03–0.05 mg/kg	
Can substitute pethidine with		
pentazocine	1–2 mg/kg	
or		
Buprenorphine	10 μg/kg	
Midazolam ⎫	0.2 mg/kg	im
Atropine ⎬	0.05 mg/kg*	
Ketamine ⎭	10 mg/kg	

*Good combinations for radiography

general anaesthesia. Well-managed general anaesthesia, with the patient intubated, breathing oxygen and regularly monitored, may be safer than deep sedation with potent opiates.

DRUG COMBINATIONS (Tables 9.5 and 9.6)

Neuroleptanalgesia is induced with a combination of an opiate and a tranquillizer or sedative. It is a distinctive state of analgesia and indifferent to the surroundings or manipulation. Neuroleptanalgesic combinations are probably the most useful in sedation for radiography.

Harmful drug interactions are a potential hazard of any combination, particularly where CNS depression may be additive. Many combinations have been shown to be safe and those which have not been tested should not be used for clinical cases.

SHORT-ACTING INTRAVENOUS ANAESTHETICS (Tables 9.7 and 9.8)

Short-acting intravenous anaesthetics can also be used for chemical restraint for radiography. These have the advantage that complete relaxation is achieved. However, in most

Table 9.7 Intravenous anaesthesia.

Propofol	Cats: premedicated 6 mg/kg; not premedicated 8 mg/kg iv Dogs: premedicated 4 mg/kg; not premedicated 6 mg/kg iv
Saffan	Cats only: 9 mg/kg iv (0.75 ml/kg) 12 mg/kg im (1 ml/kg)
Methohexitone	Premedicated cats and dogs: 5 mg/kg iv
Thiopentone	Premedicated cats and dogs: 10 mg/kg iv
Ketamine	If used for general anaesthesia probably duration excessive for radiography. Dose according to premedication. Dogs must be premedicated. Cats— see Table 9.6

Table 9.8 Drug characteristics.

Propofol

Made up in a white lipid emulsion
Rapidly metabolized, results in fast and complete recovery and no
  hangover
Single induction dose gives about 10–15 minutes
Initially slight respiratory and cardiovascular depression (as with other
  induction agents)
Ideal general anaesthetic for outpatient radiography

Saffan

Use for cats only as it is made up in cremophor EL (induces histamine
  release in dogs)
Rapidly metabolized, results in fast and complete recovery with no
  hangover. However, there can be excitement during recovery if
  disturbed
Single dose gives 10–15 minutes
Initially slight cardiovascular and minimal respiratory depression
Some anaphylactoid reactions, effects usually peripheral

Ketamine

Dissociative anaesthetic with minimal cardiovascular and respiratory
  depression
Dogs—anaesthetic doses are convulsant and premedication is essential.
  Rather long acting, cardiovascular depression if xylazine
  premedication is used
Cats—although can be used on its own, premedication is preferred to
  prevent muscle tension and salivation. Long-acting if using xylazine
  premedication, but practical for radiography if used with a
  benzodiazepine and a drying agent, eg, ketamine, midazolam and
  atropine give heavy sedation rather than general anaesthesia with a
  duration of 20–30 min which is excellent for radiography

Methohexitone

Short-acting barbiturate
Rapidly metabolized but incremental doses will prolong recovery
Single induction dose gives about 5 min
Initial respiratory and cardiovascular depression
Recovery excitable if no premedication used
Probably too short-acting and recovery unsuitable for smooth
  radiographical examination

Thiopentone

Short-acting barbiturate
Recovery depends on redistribution of the drug away from the brain;
  recovery slower than methohexitone and incremental doses prolong
  recovery substantially
Initial slight respiratory and cardiovascular depression
Longer acting than methohexitone and better recovery, though
  considerable hangover
Can be used for radiography but its short duration of anaesthesia and
  post anaesthetic hangover are disadvantages

Table 9.9 Drug manufacturers.

Drug	Trade name	Comments
Acepromazine	ACP; C-Vet BK-ACE; BK Vet products	—
Xylazine	Rompun; Bayer	—
Diazepam	Valium; Roche Diazemuls; Roche	Not licensed for animal use
Medetomidine	Domitor; Norden	—
Morphine	Morphine sulphate; Evans Medical; Macarthys	Not licensed for animal use
Pethidine	Pethidine; Arnolds	—
Methadone	Physeptone; Wellcome	Not licensed for animal use
Papaveretum	Omnopon; Roche	Not licensed for animal use
Fentanyl	Sublimaze; Janssen	Not licensed for animal use
	Hypnorm (with fluanisone); Janssen	—
Etorphine	SA Immobilon (with methotrimeprazine); C-Vet	—
Buprenorphine	Temgesic; Reckitt	Not licensed for animal use
Pentazocine	Fortral; Sterling	Not licensed for animal use
Butorphanol	Torbutrol; C-Vet	Licensed as antitussive only
	Torbugesic; C-Vet	Licensed in horses only
Alfentanyl	Rapifen; Janssen	Not licensed for animal use
Midazolam	Hypnovel; Roche	Not licensed for animal use
Ketamine	Vetalar; Parke Davis Ketaset; C-Vet	—
Propofol	Rapinovet; Coopers	—
Alphaxolone/ alphadolone	Saffan; Glaxovet	Not licensed for dogs
Methohexitone	Brietal; Elanco	—
Thiopentone	Intraval; RMB	—

cases this will only induce a few minutes' anaesthesia and incremental doses may prolong recovery unduly. Inhalation anaesthesia is probably the best for lengthy procedures that require general anaesthesia, such as angiography.

CHAPTER 10

Diagnostic Ultrasound in Small Animals

FRANCES BARR

INTRODUCTION (Fig. 10.1)

Ultrasound is defined as sound waves of frequencies greater than those audible to the human ear, ie, >20,000 Hz.

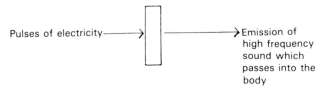

Pulses of electricity⟶ ⟶Emission of high frequency sound which passes into the body

Transducer crystal deforms due to the piezo-electric effect

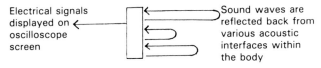

Electrical signals displayed on oscilloscope screen ← Sound waves are reflected back from various acoustic interfaces within the body

Returning echoes are sensed by the crystal and converted into electrical signals, again due to the piezo-electric effect

Fig. 10.1
How the transducer works.

Diagnostic ultrasound usually employs sound waves of frequencies between 1 and 10 MHz.

The ultrasound transducer, or scanner, contains one or more crystals with piezo-electric properties. When electrically stimulated, the crystal becomes deformed and consequently emits sound waves of a characteristic frequency. When the transducer is placed in contact with the surface of the body, the sound waves travel through the tissues. Interfaces between tissues of differing acoustic impedance reflect part or all of the beam back towards the transducer. The returning echoes are received by the same crystal and converted by means of the piezo-electric effect into electrical signals, which are analysed according to the strength and depth of reflection, and displayed on an oscilloscope screen.

There are several ways of displaying the electrical signals received (Fig. 10.2).

A mode. This is a simple method characterized by a single line on the screen. The horizontal axis represents distance and the vertical axis represents the strength of the returning echo. This is now rarely used.

B mode. Many scan lines are emitted sequentially by a single moving crystal or an array of crystals. A two-dimensional image representing a slice through the body in the plane of the beam is built up. In this instance, the strength of the returning echo is shown by the brightness of the spot on the screen. In "real-time" scanning, the image produced is continuously updated to allow movement to be seen. Real-time scanning is the most commonly used technique in medical and veterinary ultrasound.

M mode. This is an adaptation of real-time scanning. A cursor allows selection of one line on the B mode scan. In isolation this would be shown as a single vertical line composed of dots of varying brightness representing the interfaces crossed. This vertical line is, however, continuously updated and the image is moved along a horizontal axis, thus showing movement of structures along that line. Specialized M mode transducers which emit a single scan line are also available. This technique is used only in cardiac evaluation.

The overall brightness of the image can be altered by changing the power output of the transducer. This simply

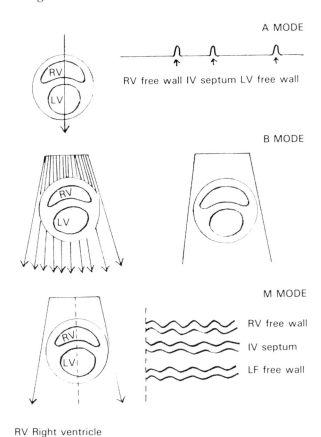

A MODE

RV free wall IV septum LV free wall

B MODE

M MODE

RV free wall

IV septum

LF free wall

RV Right ventricle
IV Inter ventricular septum
LV Left ventricle

Fig. 10.2
Consider a
transverse section
through the heart.

alters the amount of sound emitted, and consequently the amount of sound returning. Too little power results in loss of fine detail, while too much power obliterates detail due to too many echoes. As a general guide, the lowest power which still allows good differentiation of structures should be used. The gain controls allow amplification of returning echoes to compensate for attenuation due to absorption and scatter as they travel through the tissues. Echoes from superficial structures will need less amplification than echoes from deeper structures. Thus the gain for the near, middle and far fields should be adjusted to give an even image density throughout.

EQUIPMENT (Fig. 10.3)

There are two main types of transducer available.

LINEAR ARRAY

These have crystals arranged in a line along the transducer, each producing sound waves. The sound beam thus formed is rectangular in shape, which allows superficial structures to be seen well and makes it relatively easy to analyse the anatomical relationship between them. The transducer itself tends to be rather bulky and cumbersome, which limits its use in small dogs and cats.

SECTOR

These contain a single crystal which oscillates or rotates to produce a fan-shaped beam. The small size and manoeuvrability of these transducers allow ready access to most of the thoracic and abdominal viscera even in small dogs and cats. The only limitation is that very superficial structures may not be well seen due to the shape of the beam.

In general, sector scanners are preferable for use in small animals, but linear array scanners, which tend to be cheaper, can still be useful.

The resolution and depth of penetration required determine the selection of frequency of the scanner. A higher frequency

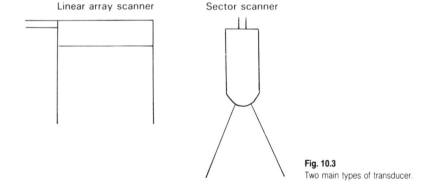

Linear array scanner   Sector scanner

Fig. 10.3
Two main types of transducer.

will penetrate less far but provide better resolution than will a lower frequency. A 5 MHz transducer provides an adequate depth of penetration for the thoracic and abdominal viscera in cats and small to medium sized dogs. A 3.5 MHz transducer is required for large dogs.

PROCEDURE

It is vital when scanning an animal to achieve good contact between the skin and the transducer. This almost invariably means that the area must be clipped, although occasionally the hair of a long-haired cat or dog can be parted rather than removed. If the skin is dirty or greasy it should be cleaned with spirit, and then a contact gel should be liberally applied. Alternatives to proprietary aqueous gels, such as liquid paraffin or vegetable oil, can be used but are more messy. The transducer is then applied to the skin surface.

If arc-shaped or horizontal white lines mar the image then skin/transducer contact is not adequate and the preparation procedure should be repeated.

Both gas and bone act as effective barriers to the ultrasound beam, as most of the sound is reflected at the surface and deeper structures are not seen. Bearing this in mind, "acoustic windows" must be found to allow the particular organ of interest to be imaged without interposition of bone or gas containing structures. There is some degree of personal preference in the window chosen, but some examples are listed below.

Heart (Fig. 10.4). Ribs and air-filled lungs act as barriers to the sound beam. Therefore the heart is usually imaged from either the right or left side, with the transducer placed in an intercostal space over the apex beat, where there is usually minimal interference from lungs. If there is significant interference from lungs, the dog may be placed in lateral recumbency and the heart imaged from the lower side.

Liver (Fig. 10.5). The transducer is placed just behind the xiphisternum and angled cranio-dorsally. The whole liver can be imaged by making sweeps from right to left, and dorsally to ventrally.

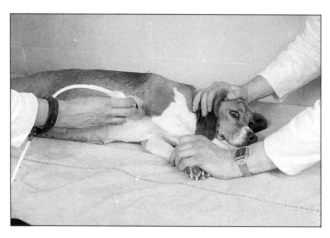

Fig. 10.4
Imaging the heart.

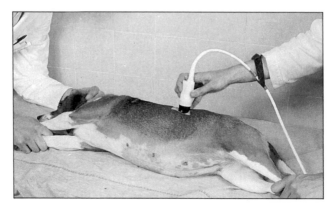

Fig. 10.5
Imaging the liver.

Kidney (Fig. 10.6). The kidneys can be imaged by applying the transducer to the ventral abdomen, but there may be interference from overlying gas-filled bowel loops. It is therefore often easier to image each kidney from the flank just below the sublumbar muscles. The transducer is placed just behind the costal arch on the left, and usually in the last intercostal space on the right.

Other abdominal organs can be imaged from the appropriate part of the ventral abdominal wall.

Occasionally variations in positioning are needed because the animal is distressed or uncomfortable in a given position,

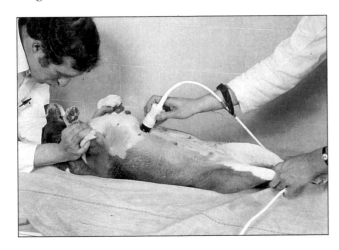

Fig. 10.6
Imaging the kidney.

or in order to displace gas-filled bowel or lung which is interfering with image quality.

PRINCIPLES OF IMAGE INTERPRETATION

The conventional display format for ultrasound scans is a white image on a black background. A number of terms are used to describe the image and some common synonyms are listed below.

Hyperechoic; echogenic—Bright echoes, appearing white on conventional scans. Represent highly reflective interfaces (eg, bone and air).
Hypoechoic; relatively echolucent—Sparse echoes, appearing dark grey on conventional scans. Represent intermediate reflection/transmission (eg, soft tissues).
Anechoic; echolucent; sonolucent; transonic—Absence of echoes, black on conventional scans. Represent complete transmission of sound (eg, fluids).

Fluid, whether free in a body cavity or contained within a viscus, is anechoic. Because the sound waves pass unimpeded through fluid, there is often a bright area immediately deep to the fluid. This is the phenomenon of acoustic enhancement and it is a normal finding.

Bone, other mineral accumulations and gas reflect the sound waves totally. The surface of the bone or gas is thus shown on the image as an intensely echogenic line. There is no penetration of sound beyond this surface, so structures deep to the surface are not imaged. This is the phenomenon of acoustic shadowing.

Soft tissues appear as various shades of grey depending on their proportions of fat, fibrous tissue and fluid.

APPLICATIONS OF DIAGNOSTIC ULTRASOUND

LIVER

The liver normally appears relatively echolucent, with an even coarse white stippling due to multiple echoes from the fibrous components (Fig. 10.7). The diaphragm is clearly seen as a thin echogenic line which moves with respiration. The gall bladder, if full, appears as a rounded, well defined, echolucent structure within the liver substance to the right of the midline. Neither hepatic arteries nor bile ducts are normally seen, but hepatic and portal veins may be visible as echolucent channels in longitudinal or transverse section. Portal veins characteristically have echogenic borders due to surrounding fat and fibrous tissue, while hepatic veins have no such

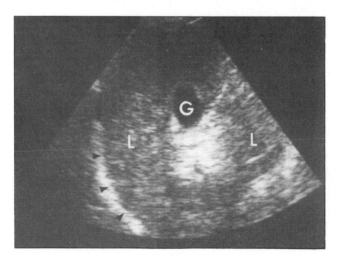

Fig. 10.7
Normal liver (L, liver parenchyma; G, gall bladder; arrowheads, diaphragm). Note acoustic enhancement (white patch) deep to the gall bladder.

border. The normal liver is slightly more echogenic than the renal cortex and slightly less echogenic than the spleen.

Parenchymal abnormalities

Focal abnormalities are readily recognized as they cause disruption of the normal uniform liver parenchyma. Hepatic neoplasia, whether primary or secondary, may cause multiple focal areas of decreased echogenicity, or a mixed pattern with areas of both increased and decreased echogenicity (Fig. 10.8). A similar picture may be seen in advanced cirrhosis. Hepatic abscesses are usually hypoechoic with thick and irregular walls or ill-defined margins. Similar pictures may be seen with necrotic tumours or haematomas. Thus ultrasound can localize the abnormality, but biopsy or aspiration will be needed for definitive diagnosis.

It should be noted that solitary echogenic patches in an otherwise orderly liver are quite common normal findings, and presumably reflect areas of fatty or fibrous tissue.

Diffuse parenchymal abnormalities are much more difficult to detect as there is often no gross disturbance in hepatic architecture, but rather a subtle change in echogenicity. Diffuse fibrous or fatty infiltration may be associated with an

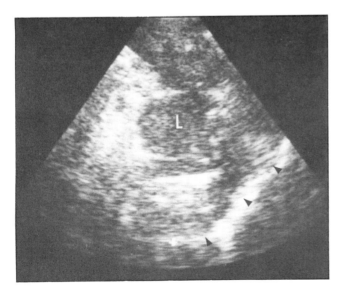

Fig. 10.8
Liver neoplasia (L, liver parenchyma; arrowheads, diaphragm).

overall increase in echogenicity. Diffuse hepatic lymphosarcoma has been associated with a general decrease in echogenicity. To assess changes in overall echogenicity it is important
to compare the relative densities of the liver, kidney and
spleen while maintaining constant gain settings.

Biliary tract abnormalities

The bile ducts are not normally visible, but may become
apparent some 3–5 days after onset of clinical icterus when
this is due to extrahepatic biliary obstruction. Distended bile
ducts are seen as echolucent channels with echogenic borders,
which have an irregularly branching and rather tortuous path.
Experience is needed to distinguish distended bile ducts from
portal veins.

Vascular abnormalities

Hepatic venous congestion secondary to right-sided cardiac
failure can readily be recognized (Fig. 10.9). Hepatic veins are
normally visible, but they become obviously distended in
this condition. Free abdominal fluid is often also present,

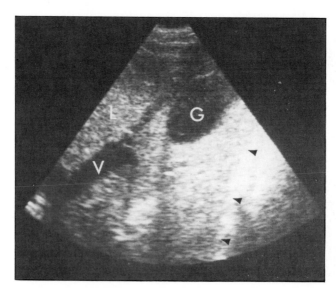

Fig. 10.9
Hepatic venous
congestion (L, liver
parenchyma; G, gall
bladder; V, distended
hepatic vein;
arrowheads,
diaphragm).

surrounding and separating the liver lobes, and lying between the liver and the diaphragm. Ultrasound can be a useful diagnostic aid here as free abdominal fluid in the absence of hepatic venous congestion suggests a non-cardiac origin.

KIDNEY

The normal kidney (Fig. 10.10) has a smooth, well-defined border. The renal cortex is hypoechoic. The renal medulla is almost anechoic and separated into multiple sections by pelvic diverticula and vessels. The pelvis is intensely echogenic due to fat and fibrous tissue.

Parenchymal abnormalities

Focal abnormalities are recognized because they disrupt the normal renal architecture. However, small abnormalities are not easily seen and in man it is recognized that solid lesions must be at least 2 cm in diameter to be imaged reliably. Renal tumours are variable in appearance (Fig. 10.11), but usually have a mixed pattern with echogenic areas relating to fibrosis or calcification, and hypoechoic areas relating to necrosis or haemorrhage. Renal cysts are well defined, rounded, anechoic structures which may be single or multiple.

Diagnosis of diffuse parenchymal disease is more difficult. Cortical echogenicity may be increased when compared with

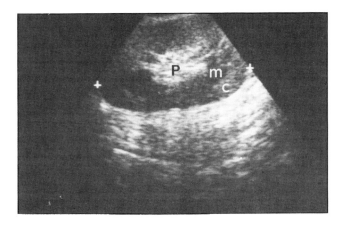

Fig. 10.10
Normal kidney (P, renal pelvis; c, cortex; m, medulla).

F. Barr

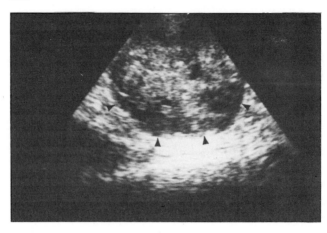

Fig. 10.11
Kidney tumour
(outlined by
arrowheads).

the liver and spleen, and there may be loss of a distinct cortico-medullary junction.

Collecting system abnormalities

Early hydronephrosis may be recognized as a scattering of the normal central pelvic echoes by an anechoic region. In more severe cases a large central anechoic area is seen with a variable amount of renal parenchyma visible around the periphery (Fig. 10.12). In some cases a dilated and fluid filled ureter is also seen leading caudally from the pelvic area.

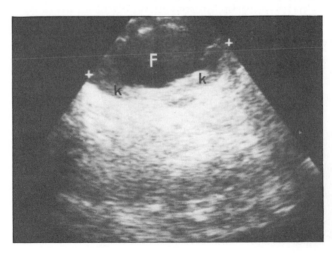

Fig. 10.12
Hydronephrosis (F,
distended fluid-filled
pelvis; k, thin rind of
remaining kidney
tissue).

SPLEEN

The normal spleen (Fig. 10.13) has a smooth contour and a uniform parenchyma which is slightly more echogenic than the liver. The multiple branches of the splenic vein may be seen near the hilus.

Focal lesions are readily seen as they disturb the normal homogeneity of the parenchyma. These lesions may be predominantly hypoechoic, hyperechoic or mixed, and may represent abscesses, haematomas or neoplasms (Fig. 10.14). Cytological or histological examination is needed for a definitive diagnosis.

Diffuse splenic enlargement with a normal parenchymal appearance may be seen in a number of conditions including congestion, vascular compromise and diffuse cellular infiltration.

PROSTATE

The normal canine prostate (Fig. 10.15) is a rounded, often rather poorly defined structure seen just caudal to the bladder. The prostate is hypoechoic with a uniform coarse stippling throughout except for a hyperechoic central portion called the hilar echo.

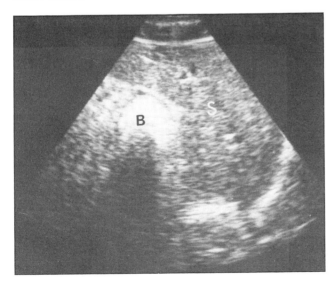

Fig. 10.13 Normal spleen (S, spleen parenchyma; B, gas in bowel, with dark acoustic shadowing deep to it).

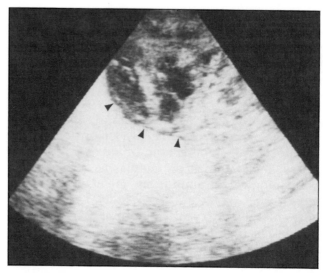

Fig. 10.14
Splenic tumour
(outlined by
arrowheads).

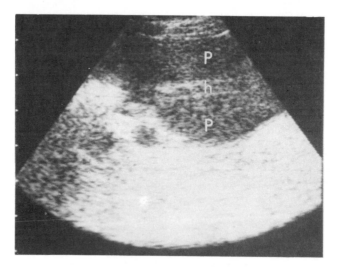

Fig. 10.15
Normal prostate (P,
prostatic tissue; h,
hilar echo).

Focal parenchymal abnormalities may be seen. In prostatic neoplasia, multiple poorly defined echogenic areas may be recognized, but a similar picture can also be seen in chronic prostatitis. Intraprostatic cysts (Fig. 10.16) tend to show as smoothly marginated and well-defined anechoic areas, whereas intraprostatic abscesses tend to have thicker and more irregular walls, and the contents may be hypoechoic

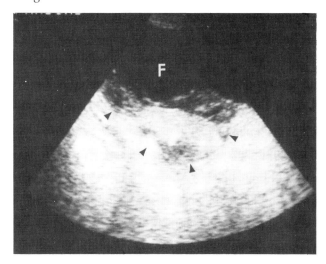

Fig. 10.16
Prostatic cyst
(outlined by
arrowheads; F, fluid).

rather than anechoic. However, for a definitive diagnosis, cytology or histology is needed in most cases.

Paraprostatic cysts have a quite characteristic sonographic appearance. They are well defined with smooth, thin walls. The contents are anechoic although internal septations may be seen.

UTERUS

The normal non-pregnant uterus is not visible in the bitch or queen. Pregnancy in the bitch can be consistently diagnosed between day 24 and day 28 after mating, when gestational sacs containing fetal tissue suspended in amniotic fluid are seen. Earlier pregnancy diagnosis may be possible in some individuals, but before the fetus is large enough to be seen clearly, care must be taken to distinguish uterus from fluid-filled bowel loops. By day 28 of gestation, fetal viability can be assessed by generalized fetal movements and fetal cardiac activity. The growth and development of the fetus through gestation can be monitored if necessary, and by day 40 fetal organs such as the liver, stomach, lungs, heart and great vessels can be identified (Fig. 10.17). The sequence of progression is similar in the cat. Pyometra is readily recognized in the bitch and queen (Fig. 10.18). A fluid-filled uterus is seen dorsal and cranial to the bladder. Echoes may be present

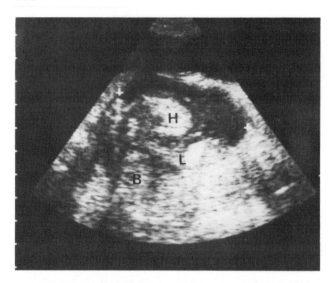

Fig. 10.17
41–43 days gestation
(H, fetal head; B,
fetal body; L, fetal
limb).

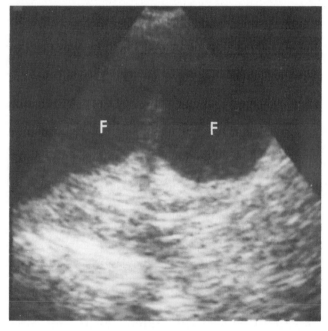

Fig. 10.18
Pyometra (F, fluid
within distended
uterus).

in the fluid if it is very thick or contains debris, but no clear fetal structures are visible.

Other abdominal masses can often also be imaged, eg, lymphosarcoma involving the mesenteric lymph nodes, adrenal masses, ovarian masses, etc. Free abdominal fluid is clearly seen as anechoic areas outlining and separating the abdominal viscera, although small amounts of fluid may be difficult to detect.

HEART (Fig. 10.19)

By imaging the heart from each side of the chest and in various planes of section, all the chambers, valves and great vessels can usually be seen. Anatomical abnormalities in these structures, whether congenital or acquired, may be demonstrated. In addition, the response of the heart to given abnormalities may be seen as chamber dilatation or hypertrophy. In real-time scanning, cardiac motion can be evaluated, and this is most accurately displayed by M mode (Fig. 10.20).

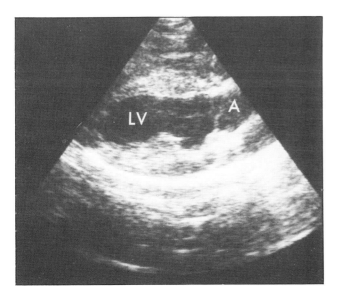

Fig. 10.19
Normal heart (LV, left ventricular lumen; A, aortic outflow).

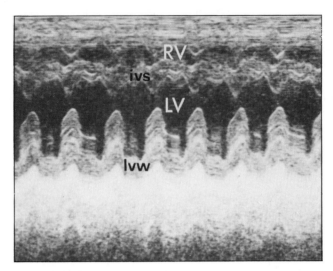

Fig. 10.20
Normal M mode (RV,
right ventricular
lumen; LV, left
ventricular lumen; ivs,
interventricular
septum; lvw, left
ventricular free wall,
including papillary
muscle). Note the
movement of an
active and normally
functioning ventricular
wall and undilated
ventricle.

Congenital abnormalities

Atrial or ventricular septal defects can be visualized if they are large enough. However, care must be taken in making such a diagnosis as apparent defects can be produced by innocent use of the instrument's gain controls.

Congenital abnormalities of the atrioventricular valves may be recognized. Characteristically there is marked atrial dilatation, although ventricular contractility is good. The valve cusps may be short and thickened with an abnormal excursion.

In aortic stenosis (Fig. 10.21), a narrowing of the aortic outflow tract can be seen, often in conjunction with a bright echo due to fibrous tissue at the site of stenosis. There may also be an obvious post stenotic dilatation.

The most common congenital anomalies, pulmonary stenosis and patent ductus arteriosus, are less easy to see, although they may be identified with experience. However, the response of the heart (right ventricular hypertrophy with pulmonary stenosis and left atrial and ventricular dilation with patent ductus arteriosus) can be demonstrated.

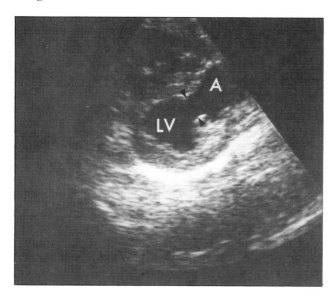

Fig. 10.21
Aortic stenosis (LV,
small left ventricular
lumen; and thickened
ventricular lumen,
and thickened
ventricular wall; A,
widened aortic
outflow; arrowheads,
point of narrowing).

Acquired abnormalities

A useful application of ultrasound lies in its ability
to distinguish between congestive cardiomyopathy and
valvular insufficiency in the dog. In congestive cardiomyopathy (Figs 10.22 and 10.23) there is generally atrial and

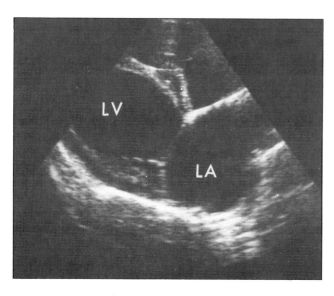

Fig. 10.22
Cardiomyopathy (LV,
dilated left ventricle;
LA, dilated left
atrium).

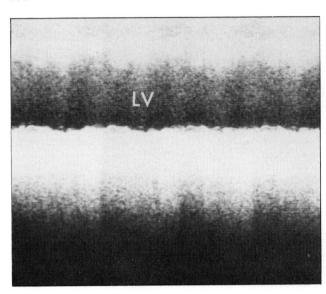

Fig. 10.23
Cardiomyopathy M
mode (LV, dilated
and hypokinetic left
ventricular lumen).

ventricular dilatation. Myocardial contractility is poor and
often incoordinated due to the dysrhythmias that frequently
accompany myocardial disease. Insufficiency of the atrioventricular valves may also lead to atrial dilatation, but
ventricular motility is usually normal, except in very
advanced cases. This has important consequences in planning therapy.

Ultrasound can differentiate between the congestive
(dilatation of heart chambers, poor motility) and hypertrophic
(increased thickness of left ventricular wall and interventricular
septum) forms of cardiomyopathy in the cat and dog.

Bacterial endocarditis may give rise to bright irregular
echoes on the heart valves.

Pericardial effusion is easily demonstrated with ultrasound (Fig. 10.24). An echolucent band is seen surrounding
the heart, the width of the band reflecting the amount of
fluid present. When the pericardial fluid is secondary to a
neoplasm, the mass itself may be seen within the pericardial
space and sometimes extending into the heart chambers.

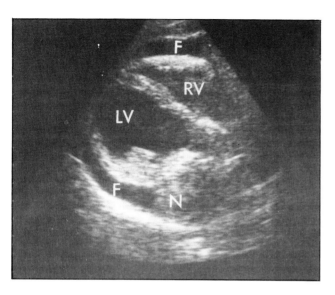

Fig. 10.24
Pericardial effusion
(RV, right ventricular
lumen; LV, left
ventricular lumen; F,
pericardial fluid; N,
heart base
neoplasm).

GENERAL THORAX

Free pleural fluid can be identified ultrasonographically as an anechoic space not related to the contours of the heart. Intrathoracic masses may be visualized if there is no air-filled lung acting as a barrier between the mass and the chest wall. Diaphragmatic rupture may be inferred from the presence of abdominal viscera, particularly liver, within the thoracic cavity. However, care must be taken in making such a diagnosis when imaging the cranial abdomen because the highly reflective interface between air-filled lung and the diaphragm commonly gives rise to reverberations and the so-called mirror image artefact. This results in liver echoes beyond the diaphragm in the chest cavity. If abdominal viscera are still seen within the thoracic cavity when imaging from the chest wall, the diagnosis may be confirmed.

CONCLUSION

In summary, ultrasound is a safe, non-invasive procedure which allows the internal architecture of abdominal and thoracic organs to be examined, and movement of structures, in particular the heart, to be evaluated. Where appropriate, it allows accurate placement of needles for tissue or fluid sampling to enable a definitive diagnosis to be made. Ultrasound is a technique which lends itself to sequential examination and so allows progression or resolution of a lesion to be followed and the response to therapy monitored.

ACKNOWLEDGEMENTS

I would like to thank all my colleagues in the Departments of Veterinary Medicine and Surgery for their cooperation in the ultrasound examination of their cases, and in particular Dr C. Gibbs and Dr P. Wotton who carried out some of the examinations illustrated in this article. The illustrations were prepared by Mr J. Conibear and Mr M. Parsons. Several figures are reproduced by kind permission of the editors of *The Veterinary Annual*. I would also like to acknowledge the financial support provided by the Alison Alston Canine Award and the BSAVA Clinical Studies Trust Fund.

FURTHER READING

Veterinary Clinics of North America: Small Animal Practice. Diagnostic Ultrasound, November 1985.
Bondestari, S., Alitalo, I. & Karkainen, M. (1983) *Journal of Small Animal Practice* **24**, 145.

CHAPTER 11

Blood Sampling in the Dog and Cat

MARK PATTESON AND PAUL WILLIAMS

INTRODUCTION

Laboratory investigations are being used increasingly by practitioners as a diagnostic tool. Properly collected blood samples are essential to minimize handling artefacts and stress to the patient.

Although many practitioners will be experienced in techniques of venepuncture in dogs and cats, this article outlines suggestions for methods of blood collection that may be found most useful. The choice of technique will depend on personal preference and individual situation. The jugular and cephalic veins are most frequently used and Table 11.1 lists some advantages of each.

PREPARATION

For most purposes the animal should be starved for 12 h before sampling to reduce the risk of lipaemia and the effects of recent feeding on blood parameters such as urea and glucose. Stress can have an effect on the blood picture, as splenic contraction causes a sudden release of stored cells.

Table 11.1 Advantages of cephalic and jugular venepuncture.

Cephalic

Familiarity with venepuncture of this vein
Some animals may be more easily restrained, especially fractious cats
The vein may be more easily seen
Intravenous injections are more easily made into this vein following
  sampling

Jugular

A large volume of blood may be obtained more rapidly
Some animals may be more easily restrained
Useful in chondrodystrophic dogs, small puppies and kittens
Useful in animals with circulatory collapse
Spares cephalic veins for catheterization

The fur over the site of venepuncture should be clipped over a large enough area to make the course of the vein easily visible. Heavy soaking with surgical spirit is an alternative in the show animal if clipping is not permitted. Electric clippers allow better and neater exposure, but they should be switched on at some distance to the animal. They may distress some patients sufficiently to preclude their use.

Frustration can be avoided by having the correct sample containers close to hand. Containers with anticoagulant should be filled to exactly the level indicated particularly for haematology. Overfilling can lead to clot formation and underfilling can alter cell size and morphology. A 0.5 ml paediatric EDTA container will normally suffice for a full haematological examination.

The application of excessive suction can cause collapse of the vein, slow blood flow and cause haemolysis. To help to avoid this the smallest syringe necessary for the sample volume required should be used and gentle, intermittent pressure applied.

In the dog we find 21 g needles are most suitable, while 23 g needles are preferred for cats and 25 g needles may be used in kittens. These smaller sizes are less likely to damage the vein which could hamper further sampling.

The length of needle used ($\frac{1}{2}$, $\frac{5}{8}$ or 1 inch) is very much a matter of personal preference. We prefer to use the longest

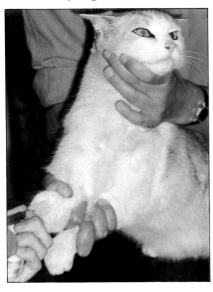

Fig. 11.1
Minimal restraint is advisable. The free leg may be held by the handler.

needle that can be threaded up the vein to the hilt and, therefore, for small dogs and cats a $\frac{5}{8}$ inch needle is preferred.

CEPHALIC SAMPLING (Figs 11.1–11.3)

For cephalic bleeding, firm handling should be used in the dog, but minimal restraint is advisable initially for most cats. Some cats need firm restraint but the majority respond better to gentle handling. This will avoid the effects of stress on the haemogram as mentioned earlier.

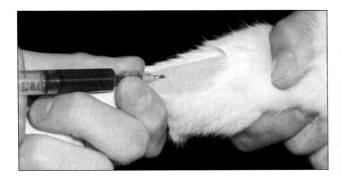

Fig. 11.2
The barrel or needle hub may be held between thumb and index finger leaving other fingers free to gently massage the paw. A wad of cotton wool can be useful to protect the palm from the cat's claw.

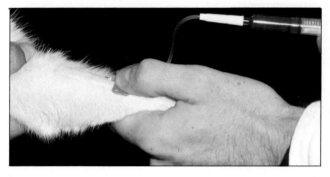

Fig. 11.3
A mini vein set may
be useful where
larger quantities of
blood are needed or
an intravenous
injection is to be
made.

The animal is held gently under the chin and the head turned away from the person collecting the blood sample. From this position it is relatively easy to "scruff" a cat if necessary. The handler's body or a wall may be used to stop the animal backing away. The really fractious cat can be further restrained by wrapping in a blanket or a laboratory coat.

Two or 3 ml of blood should be sufficient for routine biochemistry. Where greater quantities are required, or an intravenous injection is to follow sampling, a mini-vein set may prove useful to allow blood collected to be emptied from the syringe at intervals. Using these sets it is sometimes possible to collect sufficient volumes of blood for a transfusion, but they are an additional expense.

JUGULAR SAMPLING (Figs 11.4–11.8)

Animals may be held upright or in dorsal recumbency for jugular sampling. In the upright position the head is held turned and lifted away from the collector. In cats or small dogs the front legs may be grasped firmly by the handler and held extended over the edge of a table. Larger dogs may be restrained around the front of the chest. The thumb occludes the vein at the thoracic inlet and gentle tension is applied to the skin with the fingers. Raising and releasing the vein may help make its position more obvious and even if the vein cannot be seen it may be palpable. Damage to nearby vital structures rarely if ever proves a problem. The syringe may be stabilized by resting it against the thumb.

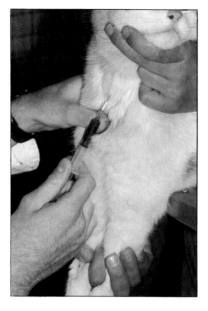

Fig. 11.4
Firm but gentle restraint is used to stop the animal
moving.

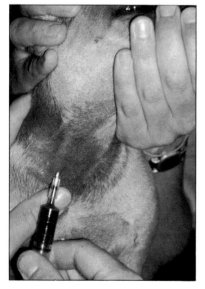

Fig. 11.5
The dog's head is turned away from the collector. The
fingers spread the skin to eliminate any folds.

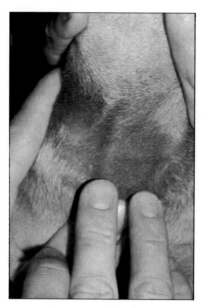

Fig. 11.6
The jugular vein is occluded at the thoracic inlet.

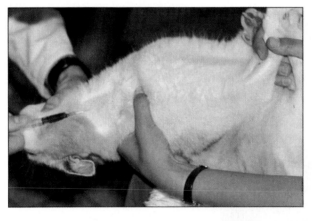

Fig. 11.7
Handler occluding the jugular vein.

For cats and small puppies restraint in dorsal recumbency may be used. The animal is placed in the handler's lap and all four legs grasped within one hand. The handler or the collector may occlude the vein. This method should not be used in the dyspnoeic animal.

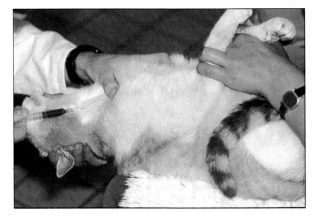

Fig. 11.8
Sample collector
occluding the jugular
vein.

ALTERNATIVES

In the dog the saphenous vein may also be used for sampling, however, many practitioners find the mobility of this vein makes venepuncture difficult. Where only a very small quantity of blood is needed from cats the marginal ear vein may be used (Figs 11.9 and 11.10). Using this method blood may be obtained for blood smears and for determining the PCV, WBC (by pipette method) and for dipstick tests only requiring one to two drops blood, eg, Ames Azostix.

The handling of the animal is of crucial importance for all of these techniques. Trained handlers enable the collector to

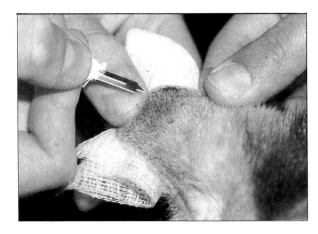

Fig. 11.9
The ear is smeared in
petroleum jelly to prevent
blood spreading. A lancet
or scalpel blade is used
to make a stab incision in
the vein.

M. W. Patteson and P. D. Williams

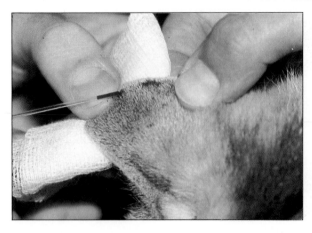

Fig. 11.10
Heparinized capillary
tubes must be used.

be confident that the animal is correctly restrained and reduces
the stress in the patient.

CHAPTER 12

Bone Marrow Aspiration and Biopsy in Dogs and Cats

JOHN DUNN

INTRODUCTION

The diagnostic and prognostic value of a bone marrow aspirate or biopsy depends on the proper collection and handling of an adequate specimen. It is also limited by the skills of the person interpreting the smears or histological sections. A detailed discussion on bone marrow evaluation is outwith the scope of this article and readers are advised to seek the advice of an experienced clinical pathologist wherever possible.

INDICATIONS

Specific indications for bone marrow evaluation are most frequently derived from the results of a full routine haematological examination. It should be emphasized, however, that haematological findings should always be assessed in conjunction with other clinical, biochemical or radiological abnormalities; for example, there is little point in performing a bone marrow aspirate when an anaemia is associated with some other primary metabolic disorder such as chronic renal failure or hypoadrenocorticism.

Indications for bone marrow evaluation include:

(1) Non-regenerative anaemia
(2) Persistent neutropenia or thrombocytopenia
(3) Pancytopenia or any combination of the above two
(4) Unexplained leucocytosis, polycythaemia or thrombocytosis
(5) Excessive numbers of immature erythroid or myeloid cells or cells with atypical morphology on a peripheral blood smear (eg, myeloproliferative or lymphoproliferative disease, or myelodysplasia)
(6) Multicentric lymphosarcoma
(7) Unexplained intermittent or sustained pyrexia, ie, true fever of unknown origin
(8) Hyperproteinaemia associated with a monoclonal or polyclonal gammopathy
(9) Unexplained hypercalcaemia

Hyperproteinaemia, especially hypergammaglobulinaemia, although rare in dogs, is a relatively consistent feature of plasma cell myelomas, or less frequently, functional B-cell lymphomas.

The most common cause of hypercalcaemia in dogs is that associated with malignancy, in particular, lymphosarcoma. One recent study showed that dogs with multicentric lymphoma which were hypercalcaemic were more likely to have bone marrow involvement (Madewell 1986). Occasionally hypercalcaemia, associated with lymphosarcoma, occurs in the absence of more overt signs of lymphoid neoplasia such as lymphadenopathy or splenomegaly and in these cases evaluation of a bone marrow aspirate may reveal a neoplastic lymphoid infiltrate.

TECHNIQUES

Bone marrow may be examined by two methods:

(1) Cytological examination of an aspirated sample
(2) Histological examination of a core biopsy

Both these procedures may be performed in most animals with sedation and local anesthesia. To ensure accurate interpretation, *blood for full routine haematological examination (including a platelet count) should be taken on the day of the bone marrow evaluation* and the results evaluated in conjunction with those of the marrow.

ASPIRATION

Marrow may be aspirated from the iliac crest (medium and large dogs) or from the trochanteric fossa of the femur (small dogs and cats) (Figs 12.1 and 12.2) using a Klima or Rosenthal biopsy needle (Fig. 12.3).

To obtain a sample from the iliac crest the animal is placed in sternal or lateral recumbency. The site is clipped and the skin, subcutis and periosteum are infiltrated with local

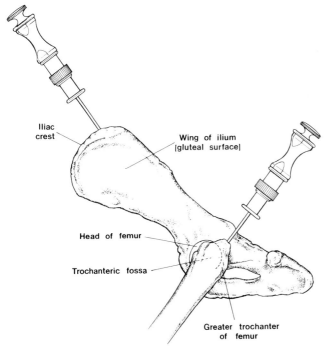

Iliac crest

Wing of ilium [gluteal surface]

Head of femur

Trochanteric fossa

Greater trochanter of femur

Fig. 12.1
Left lateral aspect of the os coxae and proximal femur showing points of entry for bone marrow aspiration.

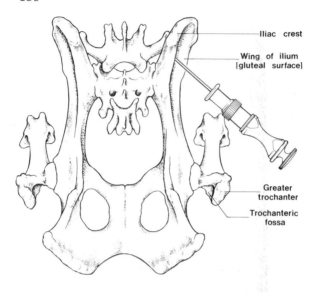

Iliac crest

Wing of ilium
[gluteal surface]

Greater
trochanter

Trochanteric
fossa

Fig. 12.2.
Dorsoventral view of the
pelvis showing point of
entry for aspirating or
biopsying marrow from
the wing of the ilium.

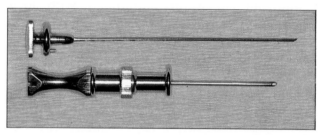

Fig. 12.3
Bone marrow may be
aspirated using a
Klima needle, shown
with interlocking
stylet; 16 gauge ×
37 mm.

anaesthetic (Fig. 12.4). After surgical preparation and draping, a small stab incision is made in the skin and the needle is advanced through the cortical bone and into the marrow cavity using alternating clockwise-counterclockwise rotations (Fig. 12.5). In doing so it is essential that the stylet remains *in situ* to avoid plugging the needle lumen with cortical bone, and that the needle is advanced parallel to the long axis of the wing of the ilium. With the needle in the marrow cavity the stylet is removed and a 10 ml syringe is attached to the needle hub (Fig. 12.6).

The marrow is aspirated by several quick, forceful withdrawals of the plunger; if this fails the needle is withdrawn slightly before suction is reapplied. If marrow is still not obtained the needle is withdrawn, the stylet is replaced and the needle is redirected. When repeated attempts to aspirate

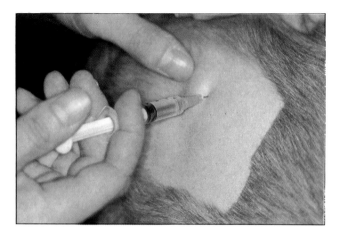

Fig. 12.4
The site over the iliac crest is clipped and the skin, subcutis and periosteum are infiltrated with local anaesthetic. The dog's back is towards the left of the picture with the left iliac crest uppermost.

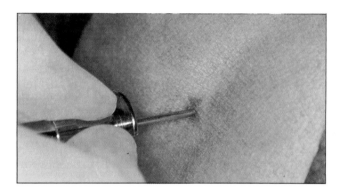

Fig. 12.5
The needle is advanced through the cortical bone and into the marrow cavity using alternating clockwise-counterclockwise rotations.

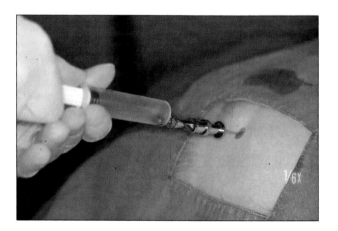

Fig. 12.6
The stylet is removed and marrow is aspirated into a 10 ml syringe.

marrow from the iliac crest are unproductive an alternative site should be tried. This involves a transverse and slightly oblique penetration of the wing of the ilium from the gluteal surface which can be palpated as a shallow depression on the lateral aspect of the bone.

When the femur is used the same preparatory procedures are adopted. With the animal in lateral recumbency care should be taken to ensure that the local anaesthetic infiltrates the deeper subcutaneous tissues and periosteum. The greater trochanter is palpated and the needle is directed medially to this into the trochanteric fossa. Once in the trochanteric fossa, the needle is advanced parallel to the shaft of the femur.

When marrow appears in the syringe (Fig. 12.7) the negative pressure is released immediately. In smaller animals the volume of marrow obtained is not great (0.5 ml or less) and continuous, vigorous suction only results in haemodilution of the specimen. Depending on the level of sedation, and assuming that the needle has been correctly placed, an animal may be expected to show a transient pain response as the marrow is aspirated. The needle is then withdrawn, with the syringe attached, and a drop of marrow is expelled immediately onto a series of clean glass slides which are tilted at an angle (Fig. 12.8). This allows blood to gravitate downwards while the marrow spicules remain at the top of the slide (Fig. 12.9). A suitable smear may be obtained by gently crushing the spicules with another glass slide which is then pulled apart

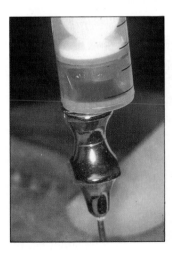

Fig. 12.7
Normal bone marrow in a 10 ml syringe.

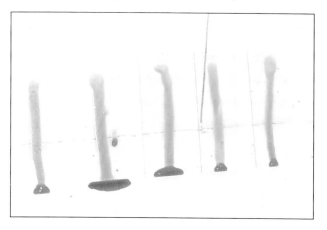

Fig. 12.8
A drop of marrow is expelled immediately onto a series of clean glass slides which are tilted at an angle. Blood gravitates downwards while the marrow spicules remain at the top of the slides.

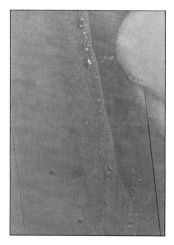

Fig. 12.9
Marrow spicules on a glass slide.

at right angles (Fig. 12.10). Smears of fluid marrow should be prepared before the sample clots (usually less than 30 s). Three per cent EDTA solution may be used as an anticoagulant. Air-dried smears which are not stained immediately should be fixed by immersion in methyl alcohol for 3 min. Romanowsky stains (eg, May-Grünwald Giemsa) are preferred for routine cytological evaluation (Fig. 12.11); staining with prussian blue will demonstrate bone marrow iron (haemosiderin) deposits.

In many cases bone marrow aspiration provides an immediate definitive diagnosis and circumvents the delays normally associated with the processing of biopsy specimens. Problems with interpretation occasionally arise when a sample is

(A)

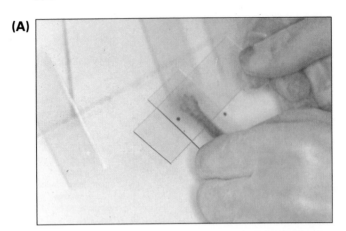

(B)

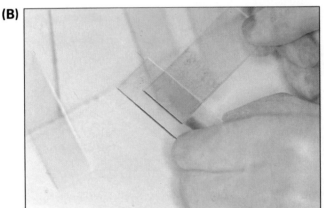

Fig. 12.10
The smear is prepared by crushing the marrow spicules with another glass slide (A) which is pulled apart at right angles (B).

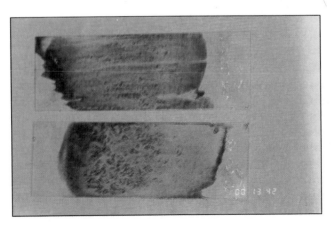

Fig. 12.11
Two bone marrow smears stained with May-Grünwald Giemsa. Note the dark blue granular deposits which represent the crushed marrow spicules.

severely haemodiluted or when the marrow is hypocellular or replaced by fibrous tissue or fat. When a hypoplastic or aplastic marrow is suspected, for example when a non-regenerative anaemia is accompanied by another cytopenia(s) or when repeated attempts to aspirate marrow are unsuccessful, a core biopsy should be performed simultaneously in the event that the aspirate is non-diagnostic.

CORE BIOPSY

A core biopsy preserves the normal architecture of the marrow cavity and provides a more representative picture of the distribution of the haematopoietic cells in relation to elements of the marrow stroma (fibroblasts, fibrous tissue, macrophages and fat). A delay in the processing time is inevitable since the specimen must first be decalcified before the sections are prepared. Cores of marrow suitable for histological examination may be obtained from the iliac crest of larger dogs using a Jamshidi biopsy needle (Fig. 12.12). In smaller dogs and cats, a transverse penetration of the wing of the ilium, similar to that described above for aspiration, using a paediatric version of the same needle has been advocated.

The biopsy needle is advanced, with the stylet *in situ*, into the cortical bone using clockwise-counterclockwise rotatory movements (Fig. 12.13). Once in the marrow cavity the stylet is removed and the bevelled cutting point of the needle is advanced gently for a further 1–2 cm using the same clockwise-counterclockwise motions (Fig. 12.14). The biopsy needle is

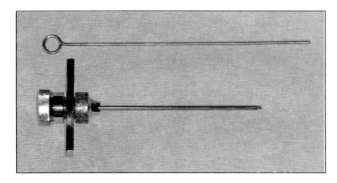

Fig. 12.12
A Jamshidi bone marrow biopsy needle (14 gauge × 95 mm). The long blunt-ended probe is used to expel the biopsy from the needle.

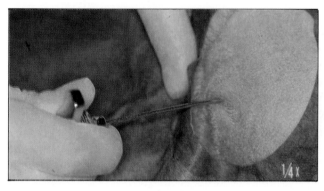

Fig. 12.13
The biopsy needle is advanced with the stylet *in situ* into the cortical bone using clockwise-counterclockwise rotating movements.

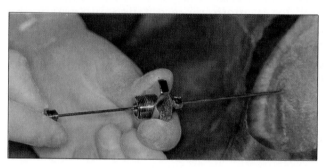

Fig. 12.14
Once in the marrow cavity the screw cap is removed and the stylet is withdrawn. The needle is then advanced a further 1–2 cm.

then rotated vigorously in *one* direction about its long axis before it is removed from the marrow cavity. To ensure that the specimen is sectioned at its base it may first be necessary to withdraw the needle a few millimetres and redirect it before removing it from the marrow cavity.

The specimen is then gently expelled with the long blunt-ended probe. This is introduced through the distal cutting end of the needle; because the Jamshidi needle tapers towards the tip pushing from the proximal end may damage the specimen.

Before fixing in neutral buffered formalin, impression smears of the marrow can be made by rolling the specimen gently on clean glass slides (Fig. 12.15).

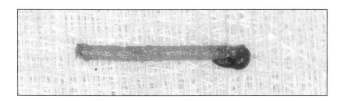

Fig. 12.15 This 2 cm core biopsy specimen is suitable for histological examination. Before fixing in neutral-buffered formalin, impression smears can be made by gently rolling the specimen on a clean glass slide.

COMPLICATIONS

There are few, if any, contraindications for performing a bone marrow aspirate or core biopsy. Problems may be encountered in obtaining a sample of diagnostic quality from very small or obese animals. Potential complications include haemorrhage, infection and trauma to adjacent structures. These problems can be minimized by choosing a superficial site and any local bleeding which occurs may be simply controlled by digital pressure, even in severely thrombocytopenic animals.

ACKNOWLEDGEMENT

Thanks to John Fuller for the diagramatic illustrations.

REFERENCES AND FURTHER READING

Grindem, C. B. (1989) *Veterinary Clinics of North America* **19**, 669.
Harvey, J. W. (1984) *The Compendium of Continuing Education* **6**, 909.
Madewell, B. R. (1986) *Journal of the American Animal Hospital Association* **22**, 235.

CHAPTER 13

Thoracocentesis in the Dog and Cat

H. CAROLIEN RUTGERS

INTRODUCTION

Thoracocentesis, or paracentesis of the thorax, means aspiration of fluid or air from the thoracic cavity. This is a relatively simple procedure, indispensible for the emergency removal of air and fluid from the chest and for the differential diagnosis of pleural effusions. In addition, removal of most of the pleural fluid allows for better radiographic demonstration of intrathoracic pathology.

PREPARATION

Animals with pneumothorax or pleural effusion are usually tachypnoeic and may adopt positions which assist ventilation. Physical examination will reveal decreased vesicular sounds and increased resonance on percussion in the case of pneumothorax, and muffling of heart and lung sounds with decreased ventral resonance on percussion in the case of pleural effusion. Radiography is required to confirm the diagnosis (Fig. 13.1) and localize the problem to one or both sides of the chest. Pneumothorax is usually bilateral, but pleural effusions (eg, pyothorax) may occur unilaterally.

Care has to be taken in handling dyspnoeic patients in radiology. Ideally, at least two radiographs, including a lateral and a ventrodorsal or dorsoventral view, should be taken, but in markedly tachypnoeic animals a single lateral exposure may suffice for initial diagnosis. Animals with large amounts of pleural effusion should not be placed in dorsal recumbency, necessitating a dorsoventral exposure. Further radiography may have to be delayed until sufficient air or fluid has been removed to permit safer handling of the animal; then, a better radiographic view of the thorax may also be obtained.

TECHNIQUE

Sedation of the patient is generally unnecessary and, indeed, might be contraindicated in severely dyspnoeic animals by causing further respiratory depression. However, especially when dealing with excitable dyspnoeic cats, manipulation and restraint can be stressful and precipitate further respiratory distress; in these patients, light sedation with a xylazine/ketamine combination may be useful. The thoracic wall should

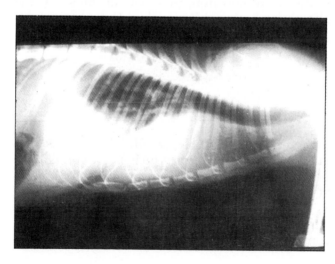

Fig. 13.1
Lateral radiograph of a cat with pleural effusion due to pyothorax.

be clipped and surgically prepared from the fourth to the eight intercostal space. If fluid and air are present in only one side of the thoracic cavity (uncommon in the dog and cat), only that side needs to be prepared for aspiration; otherwise, it is prudent to prepare both sides. Fluid is collected most efficiently in the ventral third of the sixth to eighth intercostal space with the animal in a standing position. If the animal will not remain standing, sternal recumbency (specially in cats) or lateral recumbency may be attempted. Air is collected at the highest point in the chest, ie, mid-thorax if the patient is in lateral recumbency, or the dorsal third of the chest if the animal is standing or sternally recumbent. Aseptic technique should be used during aspiration, and the operator should wear sterile surgical gloves.

Basic equipment consists of a sterile needle (1 inch; size 21–23 gauge for the cat, 18–21 gauge for the dog) and syringe (10–30 ml). Needle thoracocentesis carries a small risk of lung laceration, which is minimized by careful technique and use of the smallest size needle possible. An extension tube placed between the syringe and needle allows manipulation of the syringe without potentially damaging manipulation of the needle after it is in place (Fig. 13.2); instead a butterfly infusion set with attached plastic tubing (Surflo; Willingtons) may be used (Fig. 13.3). An intravenous polyethylene catheter (Intraflon 2; Vygon) may be used in place of the infusion set. Use of this catheter further reduces the likelihood of accidental lacerations of lungs, blood vessels or heart. A three-way

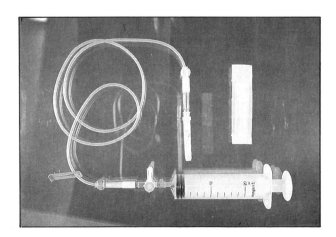

Fig. 13.2
Example of equipment needed for thoracocentesis in the dog consisting of a 21-G needle, iv extension set, 3-way stopcock, and a 10 ml syringe.

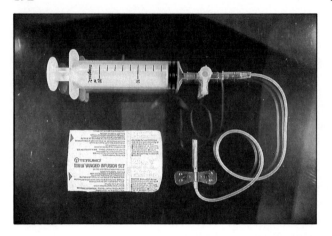

Fig. 13.3
Example of
equipment needed
for thoracocentesis in
the cat, consisting of
a 23G Butterfly
winged infusion set,
a 3-way stopcock,
and a 10 ml syringe.

stopcock is helpful if more than a single aspiration of the
syringe is anticipated. Infiltration of the skin and pleura with
a local anaesthetic may be required for the aspiration of large
pleural effusions; however, in most cases this is unnecessary.
The puncture site should always be located in the middle of
the intercostal space to avoid damage to intercostal vessels
and nerves which run caudally of each rib. Then, the needle
is slowly advanced into the pleural space at a 45° angle
with the bevel toward parietal pleura, preventing the lung
parenchyma from obstructing the lumen. Gentle negative
pressure should be applied as the needle penetrates the
thoracic wall. Advancement of the needle is stopped as soon
as it enters the pleural space, and the needle is held parallel
to the body wall, pointing downwards. Insertion of the needle
at a right angle to the thoracic wall is to be avoided to reduce
the risk of lung laceration. After insertion, fluid or air is
aspirated as necessary. As the fluid is withdrawn from the
chest, negative pressure is maintained within the thorax.
Excessive patient movement or violent coughing may necessitate needle withdrawal. Occasionally, it may be difficult to
aspirate pleural fluid even when relatively large amounts are
present, due to "pocketing" of fluid in the presence of
adhesions. In that case, the needle should be redirected
carefully while being held parallel to the body wall. In large
dogs, the needle may be held at a slightly greater angle to
the chest wall in order to increase the chance of obtaining
fluid collected in the larger interpleural space. If aspiration

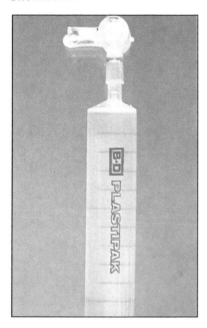

Fig. 13.4
Sample of a pure transudate pleural effusion.

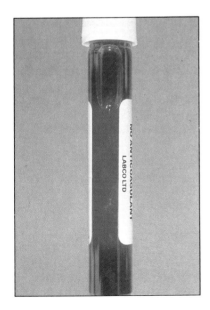

Fig. 13.5
Sample of a modified transudate pleural effusion,
obtained from a dog with a chronic diaphragmatic
hernia.

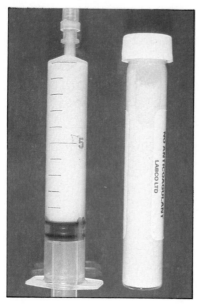

Fig. 13.6
Sample of a chylous pleural effusion from a dog with idiopathic chylothorax.

remains unsuccessful, the opposite side should be aspirated. Animals with large pleural effusions or extensive pneumothorax usually need to have both sides tapped in order to provide relief. Throughout the procedure, care should be taken to avoid air entering the pleural space and causing an iatrogenic pneumothorax. Following completion of the procedure, needle and syringe should be withdrawn as a unit. Occasionally, a slight pneumothorax results from thoracocentesis, but this usually resolves without causing problems.

Table 13.1 Physicochemical characteristics of pleural effusion.

Parameter	Transudate	Modified transudate	Exudate
Total protein (g/litre)	<30	25–50	>35
Specific gravity	<1.018	1.018–1.030	>1.018
Cells (× 10^9/litre)	<1.0	1–10	<10

SAMPLE HANDLING AND CLINICOPATHOLOGIC EVALUATION

Initial pleural fluid samples collected aseptically by thoraco-centesis should be used for laboratory evaluation. Samples should be collected into EDTA tubes for cell counts and cytology, into clot tubes for determination of total protein content and specific gravity, and into sterile tubes for aerobic and anaerobic cultures.

Laboratory examination of pleural fluid includes evaluation of its physical, chemical, and cytologic characteristics. Physical parameters include colour, turbidity, odour and clot formation (see Figs 13.4–13.6). Chemical characteristics include total protein content, specific gravity, and a nucleated cell count. Cytologic evaluation of direct and centrifuged smears is

Table 13.2 Aetiology of pleural effusions.

Transudate

Hypoalbuminaemia
  Protein losing enteropathy
  Protein losing nephropathy
  Chronic liver disease
  Malnutrition

Modified transudate

Modification of long-standing transudates
Congestive heart failure
Portal hypertension
Diaphragmatic hernia
Chylous or pseudochylous effusion
Neoplasia

Exudate

Septic inflammatory (purulent)
  Pyothorax
Non-septic inflammatory
  Feline infectious peritonitis
  Circulatory compromise (thrombosis, torsion)
Blood
  Trauma
  Coagulopathy
  Neoplasia

important in determining the cause of pleural effusion, allowing for the distinction between inflammatory and noninflammatory effusions, septic or nonseptic effusions, and whether neoplastic cells are present. Tables 13.1 and 13.2 show classification of pleural effusions on the basis of physicochemical characteristics and cytologic features.

CHAPTER 14

A Clinical Approach to the Management of Skin Tumours in the Dog and Cat

JANE DOBSON AND NEIL GORMAN

INTRODUCTION

The skin is the largest and most accessible organ of the body. Cutaneous neoplasms are diagnosed more frequently than tumours of other organs. Tumours of the skin represent approximately 30% of all canine and 20% of all feline tumours.

As the importance of neoplasia in small animal clinical practice has increased, so more effort has been invested in diagnosis and treatment. Considerable advances in the management of certain tumours have resulted from improved surgical techniques and newer treatment modalities including radiation therapy, anti-tumour chemotherapy and hyperthermia. Many tumours, particularly those of the skin, can be managed successfully if the correct diagnostic and therapeutic decisions are made and instituted at an early stage.

The purpose of this article is to present a general clinical approach to the diagnosis and management of canine and feline skin tumours. Selected tumours are considered in detail but the list is not comprehensive and the reader is referred to Brown (1985), Gorman (1986), and Theilen and Madewell

(1987) for detailed descriptions and references of tumour types.

DEFINITIONS

The skin and subcutis are composed of many different types of tissue which may be affected by a vast array of different tumours and may be broadly divided into the following categories:

(1) *Primary tumours which arise within the dermis or subcutis.* Primary tumours arise within the dermis, subcutis and adjacent connective tissues. Primary tumours can either be malignant or benign and can occur as solitary or multiple lesions.
(2) *Secondary tumours which arise at a distant site and metastasize to the skin.* These are tumours which are part of a systemic malignant neoplastic condition. These may present as solitary or multiple lesions.

Thus tumours of the skin may be benign or malignant, primary or secondary and may present as solitary or multiple lesions. The classification of primary tumours of the skin along with their relative incidence are shown in Table 14.1. Skin tumours must also be differentiated from a diverse array of non-neoplastic, tumour-like conditions including hyperplastic lesions, granulomatous lesions, inflammatory lesions and developmental lesions.

CLINICAL APPROACH TO CUTANEOUS NEOPLASMS

A prerequisite to the successful management of any neoplastic condition is an accurate definition of the nature and extent of the disease. There are inherent problems in the management of cases if the clinician concentrates on the skin mass without appropriate consideration of the patient as a whole. The clinician's primary task is therefore to:

(1)   Achieve a definitive diagnosis

Table 14.1 Classification of cutaneous neoplasms in domestic animals.

Epithelial tumours

Basal cell carcinoma
Squamous cell carcinoma
Papilloma
Adnexal tumours
  Sebaceous gland tumours
    Sebaceous adenoma
    Sebaceous epithelioma
    Sebaceous adenocarcinoma
  Tumours of perianal glands
    Hepatoid gland adenoma
    Adenocarcinoma
  Sweat gland tumours
    Adenoma/adenocarcinoma
  Tumours of hair follicles
    Pilomatricoma
    Trichoepithelioma
  Intracutaneous cornifying epithelioma

Melanocytic tumours

Benign melanoma
Malignant melanoma

Mesenchymal tumours

Fibrous tissue
  Fibroma
  Fibrosarcoma
  Canine haemangiopericytoma
Adipose tissue
  Lipoma
  Liposarcoma
Vascular tissue
  Haemangioma
  Haemangiosarcoma

(Also myxoma, myxosarcoma, leiomyoma, leiomyosarcoma, etc)

Mast cell tumour

(2) Determine the extent of the primary tumour(s)
(3) Investigate the presence of local or disseminated metastases
(4) Investigate any concurrent disease

Only when the full extent of the disease and any attendant problems have been identified is the clinician able to give a rational prognosis and select an appropriate therapy.

HISTORY (Fig. 14.1)

Detailed population studies of the age, sex and breed incidence of canine and feline tumours are limited. Those available indicate that the median age for cutaneous tumours in the dog is 10.5 years and 12 years in the cat. There is, however, some variation depending upon tumour type and certain tumours, notably the canine cutaneous histiocytoma, are commonly encountered in young animals. There does not appear to be any breed predilection for cutaneous tumours in the cat. In the dog the boxer, Boston terrier, Scottish terrier, schnauzer, cocker spaniel, bull mastiff, labrador retriever, basset hound and weimaraner have all been cited as having a high incidence of cutaneous neoplasia. To some extent these differing reports reflect the popularity of certain breeds within the canine population. A higher incidence of cutaneous

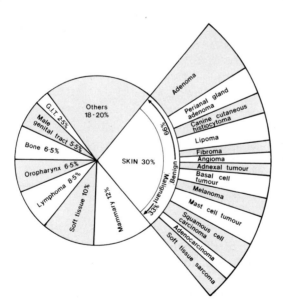

Fig. 14.1
Summary of the incidence of canine skin tumours. (Based on data from Priester & McKay (1981) NCI Monograph 54.)

tumours may become apparent in other breeds as they become more popular. For example in our clinic a large number of retrievers, particularly flat-coated retrievers, are presented with soft tissue sarcomas.

A detailed clinical history is essential. The duration and progression of signs are important. The rate of growth may be a valuable indicator of malignancy. A history of fluctuation in size might be indicative of an active mast cell tumour. Other systemic disturbances, eg, vomiting, melaena, polydipsia and polyuria must be investigated since paraneoplastic conditions such as gastrointestinal ulceration associated with a mast cell tumour or hypercalcaemia associated with an anal gland adenocarcinoma are recipes for disaster if not identified and treated at an early stage.

CLINICAL EXAMINATION

A thorough physical examination of the patient is necessary to define the clinical stage of the tumour. Whether lesions are solitary or multiple the site, extent, mobility, degree of invasion, ulceration or necrosis are all important guides to the nature of the tumour and in some cases will determine the feasibility of therapy. Careful examination of local and regional lymph nodes is important as many malignant cutaneous neoplasms metastasize via the lymphatic route. Radiographs of both body cavities may be necessary for the assessment of lymph node involvement, eg, sublumbar or presternal nodes. They are important in investigating whether or not the neoplastic disease has disseminated to organs, eg, pulmonary metastases. In the case of secondary cutaneous tumours it should not be overlooked that radiography may reveal the primary neoplastic mass.

DIAGNOSIS (Fig. 14.2)

The aim of the clinician is to define the tissue type of the mass. This can be achieved in two complementary ways: cytology and histology.

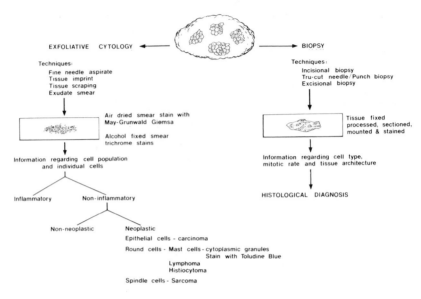

Fig. 14.2 Methods of diagnosis for cutaneous tumours.

CYTOLOGY

It is easy to obtain samples from lesions of the skin and subcutis for cytological examination. Exfoliative cytology may be performed by fine needle aspirate, tissue imprint or exudate smear. All these techniques are simple, rapid and require a minimum of equipment. Cytological examination provides information regarding the appearance of neoplastic cells and can show whether they are epithelial, round cell or spindle cell in type. In some cases, for example the mast cell tumour, this information may give a definitive diagnosis. While exfoliative cytology is not used widely in this country it cannot be overemphasized what an important diagnostic tool cytology is in the early diagnosis of cutaneous tumours.

HISTOLOGY

Definitive diagnosis of a neoplasm invariably depends on microscopic examination of tumour architecture, cell type, mitotic rate and relationship of the neoplastic cells with adjacent normal tissues. This can only be achieved by histological examination of excised tissue. Biopsy technique requires careful consideration. The accuracy of the diagnosis is to a large extent limited by the quality of the sample, and the tissue submitted must therefore be representative of the whole lesion. If the lesion is small and the site is suitable, total excision with a 0.5–1.0 cm margin of normal tissue is indicated. Excisional biopsies may also be applicable in the case of multiple lesions. Larger lesions require incisional biopsy to remove an elipse, wedge or core of representative tissue. The inclusion of at least one margin of normal tissue is essential as is adequate depth of biopsy. Severely inflamed or infected tissues or necrotic areas should be avoided as these may not provide an accurate diagnosis. The biopsy procedure should not jeopardize future treatment, nor should it predispose to the spread of the tumour. In this respect any incision or interference must therefore be made within the field of future treatment.

Histological diagnosis, clinical staging of a tumour and a knowledge of the likely biological behaviour of the tumour provide the information upon which to base prognosis and select treatment.

THERAPY FOR CUTANEOUS NEOPLASMS

The treatment modalities available for cutaneous tumours are summarized in Table 14.2. Surgery and radiation therapy are

Table 14.2 Treatment modalities.

Local disease	Surgery
	Radiotherapy
	Hyperthermia
	Cryotherapy
Local and regional	Surgery
	Radiotherapy
Systemic/disseminated/multifocal disease	Chemotherapy
	Surgery
	Radiotherapy

applicable in cases with localized disease. Where lesions are multiple or where dissemination has occurred, systemic therapy, chemotherapy or combined modality therapy must be considered.

SURGERY

Surgery is the most effective means of local therapy in general practice and is the treatment of choice for most localized skin tumours. The surgical procedure must be tailored to suit the individual case but the essential principles of good oncologic surgery apply to every case. The aim of surgical excision is to remove all neoplastic tissue. If this is not achieved local recurrence is inevitable.

Malignant tumours, particularly sarcomas, malignant melanoma and mast cell tumours, are characterized by microscopic extensions far beyond their macroscopic boundaries. The need for adequate lateral and deep margins of excision in these tumours cannot be overstated. In patients where adequate excision may seem complicated by lack of skin and soft tissues for wound closure, skin flaps or skin grafting techniques should be considered.

Effective management of malignant neoplasms depends on radical surgery. The first surgical attempt always offers the clinician the greatest potential for success (Hendersen 1986, White and Gorman 1988).

RADIATION

Radiation therapy is an alternative method of local tumour control which may be used alone or in conjunction with surgery. Ionizing radiations act upon living tissues, causing a chain of reactions resulting in chemical changes in nuclear chromatin/DNA. These chemical changes are expressed as biological damage when the affected cells attempt to replicate. Hence the biological expression of radiation-induced injury may take days, weeks or months to become apparent, depending upon the rate of cell division within the cell population. For these reasons radiation is more effective against tumours with a high growth fraction as opposed to slowly growing neoplasms, and it is not uncommon for a mass composed of non-proliferating cells to remain at the tumour site following irradiation. Radiation also affects normal tissues and those characterized by a high rate of cell division, eg, skin, gastrointestinal tract and bone marrow are particularly susceptible to radiation-induced injury. However, when used as a local treatment, radiation is well tolerated by animals and the "side effects" are usually limited to a degree of hair loss in the treated area.

Radiation facilities are not widely available for the treatment of animals in the UK but, nevertheless, this is a valuable technique which may be appropriate in cases with extensive, inoperable tumours or where complete surgical excision has not been achieved. In general the squamous cell, basal cell carcinomas and some cutaneous lymphomas are most sensitive to radiation. Soft tissue sarcomas and mast cell tumours may also be amenable to radiation therapy but tumour response may be variable according to the stage and the grade of the tumour.

In cases which present with lymph node metastases, local treatment of the primary mass is clearly inadequate. Excision of affected lymph node(s) at the time of surgery may be feasible but the tumour may have progressed beyond the grossly affected node. Local and regional lymph nodes may be treated with radiation and these nodes may be included in a treatment field prophylactically.

HYPERTHERMIA

Hyperthermia describes the use of elevated temperature in cancer therapy. This application of heat is based on the finding that malignant cells can be destroyed by exposure to temperatures in the order of 42–45°C. A variety of local, regional and systemic techniques using electromagnetic radiations or ultrasound have been developed to deliver heat to tumours in patients and this mode of cancer therapy is currently the subject of clinical trials in man and animals in many centres throughout the world. When used alone hyperthermia does not appear to offer therapeutic benefit over more conventional therapies and its main potential lies in combination with radiation and/or chemotherapy (Thompson and Gorman 1988).

Recent clinical trials using hyperthermia with radiation in the treatment of canine malignant tumours have indicated that initial tumour response and long-term tumour control may be greatly enhanced by the addition of hyperthermia to radiation therapy (Thompson and others 1987). Cutaneous tumours are particularly amenable to local hyperthermia being superficial in site and accessible for local heating.

CHEMOTHERAPY

Few cutaneous tumours other than lymphomas, mast cell tumours and transmissible venereal tumours are chemosensitive. The indications for the use of anticancer chemotherapeutic agents in the management of skin tumours is therefore limited and will be discussed in the relevant sections on specific tumour types. In each section it is not intended to cover in detail the use of anti-tumour chemotherapeutic agents.

SPECIFIC TUMOUR TYPES

SOLITARY

Neoplasms which usually present as solitary cutaneous lesions include the epithelial tumours (basal cell and squamous cell tumours), adnexal tumours, melanocytic tumours and tumours of mesenchymal origin (fibroma, lipoma, fibrosarcoma, etc). Approximately 25–35% of canine skin tumours and 75% of feline skin tumours are malignant. The general principles of diagnosis and management previously described apply to all such tumours.

Squamous cell carcinoma

Squamous cell carcinoma (SCC) is one of the most common malignant cutaneous tumours in the dog representing between 4–18% of all canine cutaneous tumours. Sites of occurrence include the limbs, particularly the digits, and the head (lips and nose). In the majority of cases the aetiology is unknown.

However, long-term exposure of non-pigmented skin to ultra-violet light can result in development of SCC, the classical example being of the pinna which develops in cats with white ears. Squamous cell carcinoma of the eyelid in cats and other species may have a similar aetiology. In dogs, the development of SCC of non- or lightly pigmented areas has also been attributed to UV light.

Squamous cell carcinomas arise from the squamous epithelial cells of the epidermis and infiltrate into the underlying dermal and subcutaneous tissues. The tumour may be "productive" forming a papillary growth with a cauliflower like appearance, or "erosive" forming a shallow ulcer with raised edges. In both instances the lesion is frequently ulcerated, infected and associated with a chronic inflammatory infiltrate. It is not unknown for these tumours to be dismissed as infective/inflammatory lesions on initial presentation.

The majority of SCCs arising in the skin are well differentiated and if adequate surgical resection can be achieved, the prognosis is good. The most malignant cutaneous SCC in the dog is that which arises in the nail bed region of the digit. This is an aggressive tumour invasion and destruction of the distal phalanx is frequent. Amputation of the affected digit(s) is the treatment of choice but these tumours may metastasize to regional lymph nodes and therefore the prognosis is guarded. Anaplastic squamous cell tumours at other sites may also metastasize via the lymphatic route, and disseminated metastases have been observed.

Squamous cell carcinomas arising on the rhinarium present a particular problem. These tumours have a tendency to infiltrate the alar cartilage and are often more extensive than may be appreciated. Furthermore this site does not lend itself to radical surgical procedures. Squamous cell carcinomas are considered to be radio-sensitive and SCC of the nose or at sites where surgery is not feasible may respond favourably to radiation therapy. One year control rates of 34–46% have been reported for radiation therapy of all SCCs (Gillette 1976) but there is considerable variation depending on tumour site and on the fractionation schedule employed. It is our experience that the tumour response rate may be enhanced by the combination of radiation with hyperthermia (Thompson and others 1987).

Soft tissue sarcomas

The term soft tissue sarcoma (STS) describes malignant neoplasms which arise from mesenchymal tissues, including dermal and subcutaneous connective tissues. Tumours of fibrous, adipose, muscular and vascular tissues and tumours arising from peripheral nervous tissues are included in this definition. In total these tumours represent 9–14% of all canine skin neoplasms. Irrespective of tissue type, soft tissue sarcomas may be considered as a group since they are characterized by common morphological and behavioural features. However these tumours do vary in their degree of malignancy and a definitive diagnosis is necessary for prognosis.

The most common soft tissue sarcomas in both the dog and the cat are the tumours of fibrous tissue, traditionally classified as fibrosarcoma and canine haemangiopericytoma. Some soft tissue sarcomas lack sufficient differentiation for definitive classification and may be described as spindle cell sarcoma or anaplastic sarcoma. A group of tumours which contain mixtures of spindle (fibroblast-like) cells, rounded (histiocyte-like) cells and pleomorphic giant cells are also recognized, some of which resemble the fibrohistiocytic tumours of man, eg, the malignant fibrous histiocytoma. As a group soft tissue sarcomas display a spectrum of biological behaviour and therapeutic response.

Soft tissue sarcomas usually develop in older animals with a mean age of nine years in dogs and cats. Fibrosarcomas have occasionally been found in dogs as young as six months old. In the cat there is a particularly aggressive, multicentric fibrosarcoma which is associated with the feline sarcoma virus and occurs predominantly in young cats less than five years old.

The distribution of soft tissue sarcomas is widespread and sites include the head, limbs and trunk. The rate of growth is variable, haemangiopericytoma and solitary fibrosarcoma may be slow growing whilst the anaplastic tumours often grow at an alarming rate. As a group, these tumours are characterized by an infiltrative pattern of growth. The tumours may appear to be encapsulated due to the formation of a pseudocapsule from compressed normal tissues. The tumour invariably extends into and beyond this structure. The treatment of choice is radical surgical excision; in most cases it is necessary to resect the entire anatomic compartments if all neoplastic cells are to be erradicated. Failure to achieve this aim accounts for the high rate of local recurrence. It is therefore essential to identify the tumour and to carefully plan the surgical procedure prior to attempting therapy. Although sarcomas are often considered to be radioresistant tumours, radiation therapy may play a role in their management, especially as an adjunct to surgical excision. Chemotherapy is usually disappointing.

The potential for metastatic spread is variable. Haemangiopericytoma is notorious for local recurrence but rarely metastasis. Approximately 25% of fibrosarcomas metastasize and although metastasis is frequently stated as being via haematogenous dissemination to the lung, in our experience lymph node involvement is quite common. The incidence of metastasis is higher in the anaplastic tumours where haematogenous spread is more common.

Other soft tissue sarcomas such as liposarcoma, and haemangiosarcoma display similar behaviour to the tumours already described. Haemangiosarcoma is a particularly malignant tumour that may arise at any site and metastatic rates as high as 90% are documented.

Melanocytic tumours

Melanomas arise from melanocytes situated in the basal layer of the epidermis or the epithelium of the gingiva. Cutaneous melanomas are less common tumours than oral melanomas but the majority which arise on the distal extremities or mucocutaneous junctions (eg, the lip and eyelid) are highly malignant. Those arising in the skin are usually benign.

Benign melanomas of the dermis are classically small pigmented nodules. Instances of spontaneous regression of such lesions are documented. Malignant melanomas may be pigmented but amelanotic forms are recognized. Ulceration and secondary infection are common features. Regional lymph node metastasis and widespread distant metastases frequently occur early in the course of the disease. It is essential that clinical staging includes a thorough physical evaluation of drainage lymph nodes and radiographic evaluation of thoracic and abdominal cavities.

Therapy for primary malignant tumours requires radical surgical excision, surgical margins of up to 3 cm are necessary to ensure complete resection. Melanoma of the extremity requires at least amputation of the affected digit, limb amputation may be necessary to achieve an adequate margin.

Some canine melanomas are radiosensitive. The combination of radiation with hyperthermia may provide an alternative means of control of the primary tumour. Prophylactic irradiation of lymph nodes is indicated if this form of therapy is undertaken. Various chemotherapeutic regimes have been advocated for treatment of malignant, disseminated melanoma but efficacy is unproven.

Canine cutaneous histiocytoma

The canine cutaneous histiocytoma (CCH) is a tumour which is unique to the skin of the dog. It is a relatively common tumour, representing up to 10% of all canine cutaneous neoplasms (Goldschmidt and Bevier 1981). There are several characteristic features: CCH is more often seen in young dogs than older animals, 50% of tumours occur in dogs under two years old. The tumours are most commonly found on the head, especially the pinna, the hind limbs, feet and trunk. The boxer and dachshund appear to be predisposed to development of CCH.

CCH presents as a rapidly growing, circular, intradermal lesion. The surface may be alopecic and is often ulcerated but rarely does the lesion cause any discomfort to the animal.

Histological sections show infiltration of the epidermis and dermis by histiocytic tumour cells with round to oval nuclei. Numerous mitotic figures give the lesion the appearance of a highly malignant neoplasm. This appearance may be misdiagnosed by non-veterinary pathologists who are unfamiliar with the condition, since the tumour resembles the human malignant cutaneous histiocytoma, a tumour which carries a poor prognosis. Despite the histological appearance and the rapid growth rate, CCH is a benign tumour which may even regress spontaneously, surgical excision is usually curative.

MAST CELL TUMOURS

Mast cell tumours (MCT) are important cutaneous tumours, representing 9–21% of all canine skin tumours. Mast cell tumours also occur in the cat and other species. The terms mast cell tumour, mastocytoma, mastocytosis and mast cell sarcoma are often used interchangeably although the two latter terms tend to be reserved for cases with systemic involvement. Mast cell tumours present a considerable challenge to the clinician and a knowledge of their unique biological aspects is essential in the management of these tumours.

Mast cells are found throughout the body in loose connective tissues and are involved in a wide variety of physiological reactions. They are widely known for their importance in type 1 hypersensitivity reactions but their primary function is related to the induction of acute inflammatory reactions in response to injury. The cytoplasm of mast cells contains granules containing numerous biologically active vasoactive peptides which include histamine, heparin, proteolytic enzymes and many other amines. It is these granules that stain metachromically to give the mast cell its characteristic appearance under light microscopy.

Appearance

Mast cell tumours may present in many guises and have been described as "the great imitator" and probably should be included in the list of differentials for any cutaneous mass no matter what its appearance. Mast cell tumours may arise in the dermis or in subcutaneous tissues, they may be solitary or multiple and internal organs (particularly the spleen and liver) may be involved. MCTs have been reported in all age groups, the mean age for dogs is 8.5 years. The brachiocephalic breeds notably the boxer, are reported to have the highest incidence of MCT, but all breeds and cross bred dogs may be affected. There is no typical appearance of a MCT but some features are characteristic. Cutaneous tumours range from well-circumscribed, firm raised plaques within the dermis, the surface of which is often erythematous or ulcerated, to poorly circumscribed, subcutaneous lesions. The tumour may be associated with inflammatory swelling and fluctuating oedema may be a presenting feature.

Histology

Many attempts have been made to categorize the clinical behaviour of MCT and to correlate this with histological criteria. Histological grading systems have been proposed recognizing three grades from anaplastic/undifferentiated to well-differentiated/mature. These grades do bear some correlation to patient survival but they are by no means absolute and in this respect the classification of MCT remains a grey area. Clinically one can recognize two basic types of MCT—solitary slowly growing tumours and rapidly growing tumours which invariably metastasize to regional lymph nodes. However, it is not unknown for a slowly growing, apparently benign tumour to suddenly develop into the aggressive variety, therefore the distinction is not definitive. It is imperative that any MCT should be treated with careful respect.

Activity

A proportion of mast cell tumours may be "physiologically" active. The release of histamine, heparin, other vasoactive amines and enzymes from the cytoplasmic granules may have local and systemic effects which are important in both the diagnosis and management of the tumour. Locally, release of histamine may result in acute inflammation, erythema, oedema, ulceration and irritation. In some circumstances these reactions may confuse the diagnosis but a history of fluctuating swelling and erythema should alert the clinician to the possibility of a MCT. Increased bleeding times may result from heparin release by tumour cells, this may occur spontaneously in ulcerated lesions or may be noted subsequent to surgical interference. Delayed wound healing may result from release of proteolytic enzymes at the time of surgery. It is because of this activity that the authors consider mast cell tumours as those that are physiologically active and those that are not. Any interference with a mast cell tumour, particularly where there has been a history that suggests that the mass has been releasing the vasoactive amines, be it physical manipulation, surgical incision or cryosurgery may precipitate histamine release from the tumour. Cases of anaphylaxis have been reported and premedication with antihistamine (H_1) agents is a wise precaution. Other systemic effects include gastrointestinal ulceration, due to chronic stimulation of H_2 histamine receptors on gastric parietal cells which results in an increased acid secretion and gastric hypermotility. Gastrointestinal ulceration must not be overlooked, it is debilitating and distressing to the patient and in severe cases duodenal perforation will occur and the associated peritonitis can be fatal. Other paraneoplastic syndromes associated with MCT include hypergammaglobinaemia and inflammatory glomerular disease.

Management

The management of MCT depends on the stage of the disease at presentation, the histological grade of the tumour and whether or not there are systemic effects associated with the release of heparin and the other vasoactive amines. Surgical excision is the treatment of choice for solitary lesions without local lymph node involvement. Excision margins of at least 2 to 3 cm should be achieved since neoplastic cells may extend into peripheral and deep tissues much farther than expected. In those instances where the histopathology shows that it is a highly malignant grade 1 mast cell tumour adjunct chemotherapy must be used postoperatively to delay the development of metastatic disease (see Table 14.3). In those cases where it is a grade 2 mast cell tumour it is strongly advised that either radiation therapy of the surgery field and regional lymph node be given and/or chemotherapy. Surgical removal of a grade 3 mast cell tumour is usually curative. Where lymph nodes are involved and/or the primary lesion is too extensive to allow adequate surgical excision, radiotherapy or chemotherapy (or both) may be appropriate but the prognosis is guarded to poor.

Any treatment which damages the tumour cells *in situ* may provoke a marked inflammatory response which will result in swelling and erythema, giving the impression that

Table 14.3 Example of the management of mast cell tumours.

Stage I	
One tumour confined to the dermis without regional node involvement	Surgical excision only
(a) Without systemic signs	
(b) With systemic signs	Where there is evidence of histamine release cimetidine 5 mg/kg every 6 h
Stage II	
One tumour confined to the dermis with regional node involvement	Surgical excision plus radiotherapy
(a) Without systemic signs	
(b) With systemic signs	Where there is evidence of histamine release cimetidine 5 mg/kg every 6 h
Stage III	
Multiple tumours: large infiltrating tumours with or without regional node involvement	Prednisolone 40 mg/m^2 daily for 14 days every other day Cyclophosphamide 50 mg/m^2 every other day may have some value
(a) Without systemic signs	
(b) With systemic signs	Vincristine 0.5 mg/m^2 intravenously weekly may also be of value Where there is evidence of histamine release cimetidine 5 mg/kg every 6 h
Stage IV	
Any tumour with distant metastases or recurrence with metastases	Prednisolone 40 mg/m^2 daily for 14 days every other day Cyclophosphamide 50 mg/m^2 intravenously weekly may also be of value Where there is evidence of histamine release cimetidine 5 mg/kg every 6 h

the lesion is progressing. Considerable effort has been afforded by oncologists to evaluating chemotherapeutic agents in the management of mast cell tumours. Despite this effort little progress has been made and it still appears that prednisolone is probably the most useful agent for systemic therapy and significant tumour regression may be achieved and maintained using the regimen based on this drug. A typical regimen is shown in the table. It is unclear what the true value of the addition of cyclophosphamide and vincristine to the treatment regimen is in the response that has been observed but some clinicians find benefit. The authors are certainly unclear of the efficacy of this combination.

An important systemic effect of mast cell tumours is duodenal ulceration. This is seen in those patients who have mast cell tumours that release significant amounts of the vasoactive amines alluded to previously. The use of cimetidine to block the H_2 receptor has proved to be invaluable in the long-term management of these cases and prevents the development of duodenal ulceration.

CUTANEOUS LYMPHOMAS

Lymphoproliferative disease is well characterized in the dog where there is a wealth of information on the various common types. It has long been recognized that the skin can be involved but the true incidence of cutaneous lymphomas in the dog remains unknown. This is largely due to the fact that the definition of the various forms of lymphomatous infiltrate into the skin is still unclear and is in need of careful examination. In this article the classification that is used is not definitive but is designed to be clinically helpful.

There are two major forms of cutaneous lymphoma in the dog that will be dealt with separately.

Primary cutaneous T cell lymphoma. In this case the lympho-cyte that becomes malignant is one that normally recirculates through the skin and is a T cell. There are two forms of primary cutaneous T cell lymphoma:

(a) Primary cutaneous lymphoma
(b) Mycosis fungoides

Secondary cutaneous lymphoma. In this case the skin becomes involved because of dissemination from a lymphoma at another site be it multicentric, alimentary or thymic. These are not all T cell lymphomas but reflect the phenotype of the original tumour.

Primary cutaneous lymphoma

The clinical presentation of cutaneous lymphoma is varied. In the majority of cases multiple lesions including nodules, plaques, erythroderma and exfoliative dermatitis are present. There is a rapid progression of the neoplasm following the initial appearance of the lesion. In the early stages dogs do not appear systemically ill but once the disease has progressed the systemic signs associated with lymphomas, particularly hypercalcaemia, are a characteristic feature. It is hard not to be impressed by the aggressive nature of this form of the disease and it is the authors' experience that the reponse to treatment is poor in comparison with other forms of canine lymphoma.

The clinical diagnosis of primary canine lymphoma can sometimes be difficult but is readily confirmed on cytological and histological examination of tissue samples. There is a diffuse infiltrate of the dermis with lymphoblasts which can extend into the epidermis.

The treatment of this form of lymphoma is similar to the treatment of other systemic lymphomas. It is folly to think that as the tumour is "simply in the skin" that the treatment needs to be less aggressive. There are a number of regimens available for the treatment of lymphoma and each clinician has their own particular one that they are comfortable with. The reader is referred to other articles for examples of detailed criticism of these drug regimens (Cotter 1986, Gorman 1986).

Mycosis fungoides

This is the epitheliotropic form of cutaneous lymphoma that is characterized by a lymphoid infiltrate into the epidermis rather than the dermis. There is a long clinical course to this disease and it is fair to say that there is no classical presentation of the disease. There are three stages to the disease: premycotic, mycotic or plaque, and the tumour stage. The first two stages can be present for many months or years before there is progression to tumour stage. In the premycotic stage there is generally a history of either an erythroderma or a generalized exfoliative, pruritic dermatitis. In this particular stage the clinical presentation can be very similar to exfoliative seborrheic condition. The premycotic lesions may have had a very protracted course before some of them progress to the plaque stage which is characterized by firm elevated plaques. In an individual animal the premycotic and mycotic stages can occur concurrently and present a very confusing clinical presentation. The final progression is to the tumour stage which is characterized by the development of multiple raised plaques in the skin. Once the disease has progressed to this stage there is usually a rapid clinical course with dissemination to the regional lymph nodes and then systemic spread of the lymphoma. At this stage clinical signs are those associated with a disseminated lymphoma.

Diagnosis of mycosis fungoides can only be achieved by a biopsy of the affected site(s). There is a characteristic lymphocytic infiltrate into the epidermis and the associated Pautrier's microabscesses. The epidermal changes also include hyperkeratosis and acnathosis but there is great variation in the severity of these changes.

The treatment of the pre-mycotic and plaque stage of mycosis fungoides has been successfully managed long-term using topical nitrogen mustard and the treatment schedule is given in detail in Table 14.4. Combination chemotherapy has been used instead of topical therapy and has overall proved to be less effective; also, in combination chemotherapy there is the added risk of systemic side-effects to the patient which can be a limiting factor long-term.

Novel methods for the treatment of mycosis fungoides are currently being evaluated. One of these is the use of 13-cis-retinoic acid which has been proposed to influence the

Table 14.4 Management of mycosis fungoides by topical mechlorethamine chemotherapy.

(1) Clip hair over whole surface of animal

(2) Dissolve 10 mg mechlorethamine (Mustargen; Merck, Sharp & Dohme) in 40–60 ml of water

(3) Apply directly to the skin. *Gloves must be worn when preparing and using this solution and the dog should not be handled for 6 h after treatment*

(4) Apply two times per week initially. Once remission has been induced treatment intervals can be reduced to weekly or every fortnight

immune response in such a manner that there is enhanced anti-tumour activity. This has yet to be verified in large controlled trials.

Secondary cutaneous lymphoma

In these cases the skin becomes infiltrated with lymphoma cells secondary to an underlying lymphoma. As a consequence of this the clinical presentation is usually one of lymphoma rather than skin disease. Where present these are usually multiple lesions and are often ulcerated.

Canine histiocytic lymphoma

It is well recognized by histopathologists that there can be a diffuse infiltrate of mononuclear cells that have a histiocytic appearance into the dermis. These histiocytic-like cells have the morphological characteristics that one would expect of a malignant cell population. However it is clear that there is considerable variation in the characteristics of this histiocytic infiltration and it is more than likely that there are a number of neoplastic diseases that hide under the guise of histiocytic lymphoma. This point will only be clarified once the exact phenotype and lineage of the cells is defined.

The variation that is noted on histopathology is echoed by the clinical course of the histiocytic lymphoma. In the authors' experience there is a predilection for young to middle-aged dogs to be affected with spaniels and collies over-represented in this hospital population. The course of the disease is generally not as aggressive as primary cutaneous lymphoma and it is the authors' impression that this group appears to be more sensitive to combination chemotherapy than other forms of cutaneous lymphoma although this does need to be substantiated.

A breed predilection for systemic histiocytosis has been reported in the Bernese mountain dog (Moore 1984). As part of this complex multiple histiocytic infiltrates are found widely disseminated in the skin with involvement of the peripheral lymph nodes. In addition, however, there can be infiltrates found in all organs. The precise nature of this particular disease remains a mystery and it is open to question whether or not this is a lymphoproliferative disease or a malignant proliferation of the histiocytic cell series. Only when sufficient cell markets become available will this be resolved.

Summary

Although the majority of cutaneous tumours are benign it is essential that a logical and rational approach be adopted for the diagnosis and management of all such tumours. The

Table 14.5 Summary of therapeutic responses of canine tumours.

	Surgery	Radiation	Chemotherapy
Solitary lesions			
Squamous cell carcinoma	Fair—good	Fair—good	N/A
Fibrosarcoma/ haemangiopericytoma	Variable Depending upon feasibility of radical resection	Fair	N/A
Malignant melanoma	Fair for local control (Depending upon feasibility of radical resection)	Variable	N/A Tendency for local and distant metastasis
Solitary or multiple lesions			
Mast cell tumour	Variable Response related to the clinical stage of the tumour and to the histological grade	Variable	Variable
Multiple lesions			
Mycosis fungiodes Premycotic stage			Topical therapy
Plaque stage	N/A	N/A	Fair—good
Tumour stage	N/A	N/A	Fair
Primary cutaneous lymphoma	N/A	N/A	Fair—poor
Canine histiocytic lymphoma	?	Unknown	Fair

prognosis in the case of malignant tumours is invariably guarded but it can be greatly improved by prompt diagnosis and adequate therapy instituted at an early stage. Surgery is clearly the treatment of choice for the majority of localized skin tumours, however, radiation therapy and cytoxic drug therapy may be appropriate in certain cases. The therapeutic responses of skin tumours to these three treatment modalities are summarized in Table 14.5.

REFERENCES

Brown, N. O. (1985) *Veterinary Clinics of North America* **15**, 46.
Cotter, S. M. (1986) *Contemporary Issues in Small Animal Practice*, Vol. 6, *Oncology* (ed. N. T. Gorman), p. 169. New York, Churchill Livingstone.
Gillette, E. L. (1976) *Journal of the American Veterinary Medical Association* **12**, 359.
Goldschmidt, M. H. & Bevier, D. E. (1981) *Compendium of Continuing Education for Practicing Veterinarians* **3**, 588.
Gorman, N. T. (ed.) (1986) *Contemporary Issues in Small Animal Practice*, Vol. 6, *Oncology*, p. 121. New York, Churchill Livingstone.
Henderson, R. A. (1986) *Contemporary Issues in Small Animal Practice*, Vol. 6, *Oncology* (ed. N. T. Gorman), p. 45. New York, Churchill Livingstone.
Moore, P. F. (1984) *Veterinary Pathology* **21**, 554.
Theilen, G. & Madewell, B. R. (1987) *Veterinary Clinical Oncology*. Philadelphia, Lea and Febiger.
Thompson, J. M., Gorman, N. T. & Bleehen, N. M. (1987) *Journal of Small Animal Practice* **28**, 457.
Thompson, J. M. & Gorman, N. T. (1988) *Veterinary Annual* **28**.
Thompson, J. M. (1986) *Contemporary Issues in Small Animal Practice*, Vol. 6, *Oncology* (ed. N. T. Gorman), p. 89. New York, Churchill Livingstone.
White, R. A. S. & Gorman, N. T. (1988) *Veterinary Annual* **28**.

The figures quoted in sections on solitary tumours and data for the table on tumours of the skin and subcutis and the figure giving a summary of the relative incidence of canine skin tumours are from:

Bevier, D. E. & Goldschmidt, M. H. (1981) *Compendium on Continuing Education for Practicing Veterinarians* **3**, 389.
Bevier, D. E. & Goldschmidt, M. H. (1981) *Compendium on Continuing Education for Practicing Veterinarians* **3**, 506.
Conroy, J. D. (1983) *Journal of the American Animal Hospitals Association* **19**, 91.
Dorn, C. R., Taylor, D. O. N. & Schneider, R. (1968) *Journal of the National Cancer Institute* **40**, 307.
McChesney, A. E. & Stephens, T. C. (1980) *Veterinary Pathology* **17**, 316.
Moulton, J. E. (1978) *Tumours in Domestic Animals*.

Priester, W. A. & McKay, F. W. (1980) *National Cancer Institute, Monograph* **54**.

Schneider, R. (1975) *A Population Based Animal Tumour Registry* (eds D. G. Ingram, W. R. Mitchell, and S. W. Martin), *Animal Disease Monitoring*. Springfield, Illinois.

Sells, D. M. & Conroy, J. D. (1976) *Journal of Comparative Pathology* **86**, 121.

Strafuss, A. C. (1985) *Veterinary Clinics of North America, Small Animal Practice* **15**, 473.

Susaneck, S. J. (1983) *Compendium on Continuing Education for Practicing Veterinarians* **5**, 251.

CHAPTER 15

Oral Tumours in Dogs and Cats

JANE DOBSON AND RICHARD WHITE

INTRODUCTION

The oral cavity is a common site for the development of neoplasms in small animals. A broad spectrum of tumour types occurs at this site, ranging from the relatively benign "epulides" to the more aggressive squamous cell carcinoma, fibrosarcoma and the highly malignant melanoma. Many of these tumours traditionally carried a poor prognosis because of their metastatic potential and the managemental problems arising through their close association with bone and the lack of mobile soft tissues within the mouth. Development of radical surgical techniques and the application of radiation therapy with hyperthermia have dramatically improved the clinical management of these tumours. This article provides an update on the clinico-pathological features of the more common oral tumours in the dog and cat and the clinical approach to their diagnosis and treatment.

CLINICAL APPROACH

Successful management of oral tumours depends upon prompt diagnosis, accurate determination of the extent of the tumour at the time of first presentation and selection of the appropriate treatment.

Oral tumours present with a variety of signs including dysphagia, halitosis, haemorrhage, displacement or loss of teeth and facial swelling. Although gross inspection of an oral neoplasm may give some indication of histiogenesis, a definitive diagnosis can only be made upon histological examination of tumour tissue. Ideally this diagnosis should be achieved by biopsy of the tumour prior to the definitive treatment. Intraoral neoplasms are usually accessible for incisional biopsy. However, care must be taken to ensure a representative sample of the tumour is collected. The surface of oral tumours may be infected or necrotic; hyperplastic or inflammatory reactions in the adjacent tissues are common and so small, superficial biopsies can be misleading. As many oral tumours involve the underlying bone a deep wedge or needle-type biopsy is recommended.

The clinical stage of the neoplasm with respect to the extent of the primary tumour, involvement of local and regional lymph nodes and distant metastases is of paramount importance in treatment selection and formulating a prognosis.

PRIMARY TUMOUR

Physical and radiographic assessment of the primary tumour is necessary to determine the extent of the tumour and involvement of adjacent tissues. Sixty to 70% of malignant oral tumours involve bone.

Good quality radiographs of the tumour site are essential in the evaluation of oral tumours. Lateral and dorsoventral/ ventrodorsal views of the skull may be useful but non-screen, intraoral films provide better detail. A variety of bony changes occur in association with oral tumours ranging from osteolysis, which may be diffuse or localized, to productive changes associated with periosteal elevation and mineralization of soft tissue tumours. These radiographic changes are rarely specific for a particular tumour type but the extent of the changes is extremely important in planning therapy.

DETECTION OF LOCAL AND DISTANT METASTASES (Table 15.1)

More than half of the tumours occurring in the oropharynx are malignant and consideration must be given to the possibility of metastasis via the lymphatic or haematogenous routes.

The lymphatic drainage of the oral cavity is primarily to the mandibular and maxillary lymph nodes. Regional drainage is to the retropharyngeal nodes and via the cervical chain to the prescapular and anterior mediastinal nodes. The tonsils should also be evaluated especially in the case of malignant melanoma. The frequent secondary infection or necrosis associated with oral tumours may lead to a reactive local lymphadenopathy. Cytological examination of fine needle aspirates taken from enlarged lymph nodes is a quick and convenient method for assessing suspect lymph nodes.

The detection of distant metastases presents difficulties. Malignant tumours which disseminate via the haematogenous route can subsequently develop at many sites including the lungs, liver, spleen, skin, kidneys and bone. The lungs are the most common site for metastases in small animals and thoracic radiographs should always be taken. It must be

Table 15.1 Behavioural characteristics of the common oral tumours.

	Epulis	AE	SCC(N–T)	SCC(T)	Fibrosarcoma	Melanoma
Local						
Bone invasion		Common	Common	n/a	Common	Common
No		>90%	>77%		60–70%	50–60%
Metastasis						
Lymph nodes						
No		No	5–10%	98%	20%	60–75%
Distant						
No		No	3–36%	>63%	27%	61–67%

Figures based on Todoroff & Brodey (1979)

recognized, however, that small tumour deposits (less than 0.5 cm diameter) are below the threshold of standard radiographic detection.

PRINCIPLES OF THERAPY FOR ORAL TUMOURS

The ultimate aim of cancer therapy is the elimination of all neoplastic cells. In most oral tumours treatment of the primary tumour is the major consideration because, with the exception of malignant melanoma, tonsillar squamous cell carcinoma and some of the anaplastic sarcomas, the more common oral tumours are slow to metastasize. Local recurrence is a more frequent problem than metastasis.

A variety of therapeutic techniques including surgery, cryosurgery, radiation therapy and hyperthermia have been used in the management or oral tumours. The choice of therapy depends upon the histological type and the extent of the tumour. The responses of common oral tumours to these techniques are summarized in Tables 15.2 and 15.3.

Table 15.2 Therapeutic response of non-metastatic canine oral tumours.

	Epulis	Acanthomatous epulis	Ameloblastoma
Surgery			
Local excision	Usually adequate Low recurrence rate	Inadequate High recurrence rate	Inadequate High recurrence rate
Wide local excision*	Occasionally necessary	Usually curative	Usually curative
Radiation therapy	Not indicated	Highly radiosensitive† Usually curative	Insufficient data
Radiation & hyperthermia	Not indicated	Highly responsive† Usually curative	Unknown

*Wide local excision = mandibulectomy/maxillectomy
†Subsequent development of malignant tumours at site of previously irradiated tumours has been recorded

Table 15.3 Local therapeutic response of malignant canine oral tumours.

	SCC–NT	Fibrosarcoma	Melanoma
Surgery Local excision	Inadequate High local recurrence	Inadequate High local recurrence	Inadequate High local recurrence
Wide local excision*	Local control of early stage tumours	Local recurrence in >50%	Local control of early stage tumours
Radiation therapy	Radiosensitive Good response	Radioresistant Poor response	Often radiosensitive Variable response†
Surgery & radiation	Good response	Decreases local recurrence rate	Decreases local recurrence rate†
Radiation & hyperthermia	Good response	Improved response vs RT only	Highly responsive†

*Wide local excision = mandibulectomy/maxillectomy
†Radiation may also be applied to local and regional lymph nodes in these cases

SURGERY

Surgical resection is the single most effective means of treatment for oral tumours. For surgical treatment to be successful the entire tumour must be excised with adequate margins of surrounding normal tissue. Since a high proportion of oral tumours involve bone it is essential that the surgical margins are achieved in the bone as well as in the soft oral tissues. The techniques of mandibulectomy and maxillectomy have been well documented in recent years. These techniques permit wide local excision of oral tumours with 1–2 cm margins of resection and have been successfully used in the management of acanthomatous epulides, squamous cell carcinoma and low-grade fibrosarcoma.

CRYOSURGERY

Cryotherapy has been advocated for use in the treatment of oral neoplasia and is well tolerated in the oral cavity. However, the role of cryotherapy in the management of the malignant oral tumours is limited because it is difficult to achieve adequate treatment of the tumour margins, particularly those within the bone and tumours often recur. Palliative cryosurgery may be used where more aggressive therapies are not feasible or appropriate.

RADIATION THERAPY

Radiation therapy has been successfully used in the management of oral tumours in the cat and dog either alone, in combination with surgery or in combination with hyperthermia. Radiation offers the advantage of treating larger areas of tissue surrounding the tumour than may be possible by surgery and high energy ionizing radiation has good penetration of bone. Local lymph nodes can also be included in the treatment fields where necessary. For these reasons the main indication for radiotherapy is in the treatment of oral tumours which by virtue of their site or extent are not amenable to surgical excision.

A number of factors govern the sensitivity of oral tumours to radiation. In general the tumours of epithelial origin (squamous cell carcinoma) are more radiosensitive than the sarcoma type. Growth rate and tumour volume also influence radiosensitivity. Larger tumours tend to be less responsive to radiation because of their slow growth rate and higher proportion of radioresistant tumour cells. Cytoreductive surgery prior to irradiation can be beneficial in such cases.

HYPERTHERMIA

The basis for the use of hyperthermia in the treatment of cancer is that malignant cells can be destroyed by exposure to temperatures in the order of 42–45°C. Radioresistant tumour cells are often sensitive to the effects of hyperthermia hence there is strong rationale for combination of the two. Hyperthermia may be induced by radiofrequency or microwave techniques and a number of clinical veterinary studies using such techniques have demonstrated that the combination of radiation and hyperthermia is particularly successful in the treatment of oral tumours.

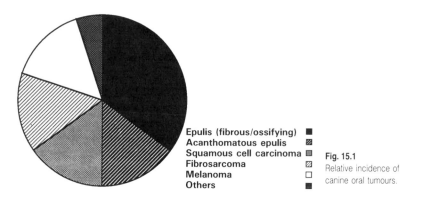

Epulis (fibrous/ossifying) ■
Acanthomatous epulis ▨
Squamous cell carcinoma ▨
Fibrosarcoma ▨
Melanoma ☐
Others ■

Fig. 15.1
Relative incidence of
canine oral tumours.

SPECIFIC ORAL TUMOURS

The approximate incidence of specific types of tumour in the
oral cavity is summarized in Figs 15.1 and 15.2. The accuracy
of these figures is difficult to ascertain as many of the more
benign tumours may not be detected or receive veterinary
attention. There also is considerable variation in the reported
incidence of certain tumour types; malignant melanoma, for
example, is reported by several authors to be the most common
malignant oral tumour (Brodey 1960, Dorn and Priester 1976)
yet, in our referral centre, malignant melanoma is 'the least
common of the three main malignant tumours of the oral
cavity (White and others 1985a).

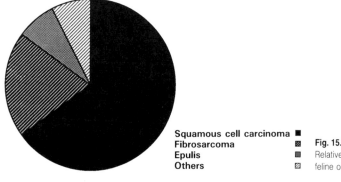

Squamous cell carcinoma ■
Fibrosarcoma ▨
Epulis ■
Others ▨

Fig. 15.2
Relative incidence of
feline oral tumours.

EPULIDES

The "epulides" are a group of common, non-metastatic oral
tumours arising in association with the gingiva. As a group
the epulides represent up to 40% of all oral tumours in the
dog. Despite this frequency there is continuing confusion
over the classification and nomenclature of these tumours.
Currently there are three systems of classification in general
usage which are summarized in Table 15.4.

On the basis of clinical and radiographic behaviour the
epulides can be considered to comprise two distinct tumour
species; the benign fibromatous/ossifying epulis (also termed

Table 15.4 Classification of canine "epulides".

Synonyms	Origin	Clinical/histological features
Fibromatous and ossifying epulis	Head (1976)	Benign lesion, slow growing, non-invasive, hard nodule
Fibromatous epulis Osseous epulis Peripheral odontogenic fibroma	Dubielzig and others (1979) Bostock & White (1987)	Comprises proliferative fibrous stroma, with odontogenic epithelium and variable amounts of well differentiated metaplastic bone
Acanthomatous epulis Basal cell carcinoma Adamantinoma	Dubielzig and others (1979) Bostock & White (1987)	Locally aggressive neoplasm Infiltration into adjacent bone Comprises broad sheets and ribbons of epithelial cells in a collagenous stroma
Ameloblastoma	Dubielzig and others (1979) Bostock & White (1987)	Always confined within bone causes gross cystic swelling and distortion Comprises broad sheets of epithelial cells, large foci with cystic degeneration

peripheral odontogenic fibroma) and the locally aggressive acanthomatous epulis (also termed basal cell carcinoma and in some cases, incorrectly, adamantinoma).

Fibromatous/ossifying epulis (peripheral odontogenic fibroma)

Fibromatous/ossifying epulis is the most common oral tumour in the dog (Fig. 15.3); it is less frequent in the cat. This tumour presents as a firm or hard mass usually with a smooth, non-ulcerated surface. It is firmly attached to the gingiva and periosteum of the dental arcade and grows outward, often from a relatively narrow base.

These tumours show varying degrees of mineralization, leading to the arbitrary distinction between the fibromatous and ossifying forms. The term peripheral odontogenic fibroma has been proposed to encompass both types on the basis that although they contain elements of odontogenic epithelium, they appear to be of mesenchymal origin.

Clinically these tumours are benign, they never invade the adjacent bone and they never metastasize. The treatment of choice is local surgical excision. Resection of alevolar bone at the base of the mass may be necessary to effect a complete removal, but the prognosis is excellent.

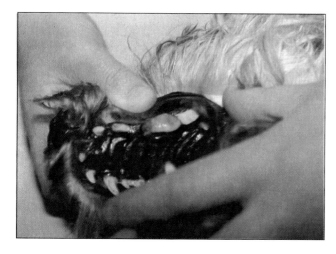

Fig. 15.3
Fibromatous epulis arising in the left maxilla.

Acanthomatous epulis (basal cell carcinoma)

While less common than the fibromatous/ossifying epulis, the acanthomatous epulides still represent a sizeable proportion of all canine oral tumours. In contrast to the fibromatous epulis, the acanthomatous epulis is a locally aggressive tumour and it invariably invades the adjacent alveolar bone.

The gross appearance of this tumour is variable. It may present as an irregular, fungating epithelial mass or it may be more invasive, with an ulcerated appearance and occasionally it contains extensive areas of necrosis. Radiographically, there is usually lysis of adjacent alveolar bone and displacement or loss of teeth is common (Fig. 15.4). Occasionally, the soft tissue of the tumour becomes mineralized.

The term basal cell carcinoma has been applied to this tumour, on the basis that the lesion is predominantly composed of clumps of epithelium attached to and apparently originating from the stratum germanitivum of the overlying gum. The consistent infiltration into bone is characteristic of the behaviour of a carcinoma.

Although acanthomatous epulis does not metastasize, it does present a clinical problem by virtue of the invasive pattern of growth. Simple local excision with minimal tumour margins is rarely sufficient to prevent local recurrence. The treatment of choice is wide local excision, including a margin of at least 1 cm of alveolar bone beyond the radiographic limit of the tumour. This surgical approach has been shown to be effective in achieving a local cure in a high percentage of cases.

Acanthomatous epulides are extremely sensitive to radiation and high cure rates can also be achieved by radiotherapy. However, surgery is the preferred treatment because there is a risk of the subsequent development of malignant tumours at the site of irradiated acanthomatous epulides.

Ameloblastoma

Ameloblastoma is a rare tumour which arises in association with the dental enamel-forming organ (Rests of Mallasez). It characteristically occurs in young animals. In dogs the

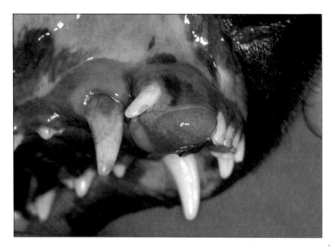

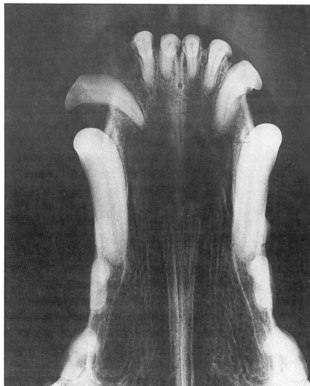

Fig. 15.4
Acanthomatous
epulis involving the
premaxilla.
Displacement of the
third incisor and
mineralization at the
centre of the soft
tissue mass is shown
on the radiograph.

234 J. M. Dobson and R. A. S. White

mandible is the usual site (Fig. 15.5), whereas ameloblastoma appears to be more frequent in the maxilla of cats. At either site, the expansile growth of the tumour results in gross swelling and distortion of the bone. The tumour is composed of well-defined, large cystic cavities and thus has a characteristic loculate radiographic appearance. In our experience, these tumours can be cured by complete surgical resection.

(In humans the term "adamantinoma" is used synonymously with "ameloblastoma". In the veterinary literature adamantinoma has also been used to describe acanthomatous epulis.

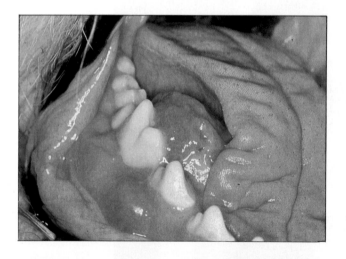

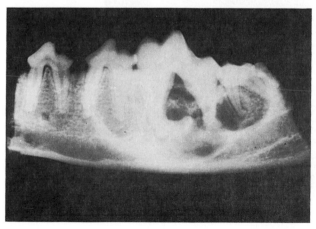

Fig. 15.5
Ameloblastoma of the mandibular ramus with typical cystic swelling originating in the bone. Radiographic changes are characteristic.

Because of the confusion this may cause, we suggest that the term adamantinoma should be abandoned.)

SQUAMOUS CELL CARCINOMA (Fig. 15.6)

Squamous cell carcinoma (SCC) is the most common malignant oral tumour in the dog and cat. Oropharyngeal SCC may be

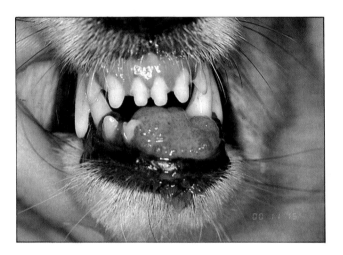

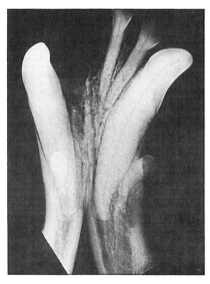

Fig. 15.6
Squamous cell carcinoma of the mandibular symphysis. The incisor teeth have been lost and lysis of the symphyseal bone is evident radiographically.

divided into tonsillar SCC, soft tissue (ie, lingual and labial) SCC and gingival SCC for descriptive and prognostic purposes.

Gingival SCC

Gingival SCC may arise at any site in the upper and lower dental arcades and it usually affects middle-aged to elderly animals. There is no apparent breed or sex predilection in either species. The tumour usually begins at the gingival margin and its invasive growth leads to destruction of the periodontal tissues and loosening of the teeth. The gross appearance is of an irregular, proliferative or ulcerative epithelial lesion. The tumour is often friable and haemorrhagic, and secondary bacterial infection is common. Invasion and lysis of adjacent bone occurs in over 70% of cases.

As gingival SCC has a low rate of metastasis, the major managemental priority is control of the primary tumour. Surgery is the treatment of choice for early stage lesions, particularly those affecting rostral areas of the mouth. Wide local excision by maxillectomy or mandibulectomy, as appropriate, is frequently curative, and one year survival rates are in the order of 90%. SCC is radiosensitive and radiotherapy is indicated for more advanced tumours or those involving sites where surgery is not feasible. The combination of radiation and hyperthermia has proved particularly effective in the management of some of the more advanced tumours.

Soft tissue (labial and lingual) SCC

SCC may also arise in the soft tissues of the lips and tongue. The frenulum of the tongue was reported to be one of the most common sites for SCC in urban cats and although the incidence may now have decreased, this is still an important site in this species. The incidence of lingual SCC in dogs is considerably lower, representing perhaps 5–10% of all oropharyngeal SCC.

SCC of the tongue is a particularly aggressive neoplasm which is characterized by rapid extension and invasion into the tongue. The tumour often involves the full thickness of the tongue by the time of presentation. The lesion is frequently painful, resulting in difficulties in prehension and mastication, excessive salivation (often purulent or blood-tinged) and halitosis. Lymphatic invasion and spread are common. The lingual form presents particular managemental problems: the extensive infiltration of the tongue often precludes effective surgical resection and although the tumour is usually radiosensitive, normal tissue tolerance at this site is poor and the therapeutic index is low.

On occasion SCC arises in the epithelium of the mucosal surface of the lip or cheek. Tumours at this site are often more ulcerative than proliferative in nature and may initially be mistaken for oral ulceration. SCC of the lip is not generally as aggressive as the lingual form but the lesion is often acutely painful to the animal. Wide local surgical resection is the treatment of choice and radiotherapy may also be appropriate in some cases.

Tonsillar SCC

Tonsillar SCC is less common than the gingival form, but there is considerable regional variation in the reported incidence and it appears that this form of the disease may have been more common in the past (particularly in animals living in cities) than it is now. In the dog the average age of onset of the disease is nine to 10 years and males are affected three times more than bitches. SCC of the tonsil is rare in the cat.

Tonsillar SCC usually presents as a unilateral lesion, although bilateral involvement has been reported. In early cases the tonsil is of relatively normal size but shows a number of small papillomatous growths on its surface. Infiltration and destruction of the tonsil develop rapidly and the tumour progresses to involve the pharyngeal wall and soft palate. This lesion is often acutely painful and affected animals present with symptoms of dysphagia, difficulty in swallowing, gagging, hypersalivation and weight loss.

SCC of the tonsil is an aggressive tumour and the incidence of metastasis to the retropharyngeal lymph nodes is high. Haematological dissemination may also occur. Occasionally the first manifestation of the disease is an enlarged retropharyngeal lymph node. By virtue of its rapid local progression and high rate of metastasis, the prognosis for tonsillar SCC is poor. The results of therapy either by surgical resection, radiation or combinations of the two are usually disappointing and median survival times are in the region of two months.

FIBROSARCOMA

Fibrosarcoma is the second most common malignant tumour of the canine oropharynx. It tends to occur in younger dogs, the mean age of onset is 7.5 years but up to 25% occur in animals under five years. There is a 2:1 male:female ratio and in our experience the retriever breeds appear to suffer a particularly high incidence of oral fibrosarcoma. Although fibrosarcoma is a common tumour in the cat, its incidence in the oral cavity is low, sites of predilection being the soft tissues of the head, trunk and limbs.

In the dog, oral fibrosarcoma most commonly involves the upper dental arcade, often extending dorsally into the paranasal region and medially into the palate (Fig. 15.7). The ramus of the mandible is also frequently affected. Fibrosarcoma usually presents as a firm, smooth mass with a broad base and in its early stages it may not easily be distinguished on gross inspection from gingival hyperplasia or fibromatous epulis. Radiographic evidence of bone involvement is common in more advanced tumours, but in general fibrosarcoma tends

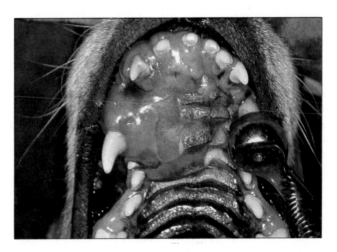

Fig. 15.7
Fibrosarcoma of the premaxilla. Note the extent of the tumour in the incisor region, with marked displacement of the incisor teeth.

to cause less lysis than SCC or acanthomatous epulis and it is more often associated with a proliferative periosteal reaction. Local and distant metastases occur in around 25% of cases, but the prognosis is always guarded due to the extensive infiltration of adjacent tissues. No single form of treatment has been found to be entirely effective in eradication of oral fibrosarcoma. Wide local surgical excision by mandibulectomy and maxillectomy may control early stage, low grade tumours, but even such aggressive surgery does not achieve the compartmental type of resection which is necessary to eradicate most oral fibrosarcomas. Fibrosarcoma is not particularly sensitive to radiation and radiotherapy alone does not appear to offer any significant improvement in local tumour control over surgery.

The most successful approaches to the treatment of oral fibrosarcoma have been through combined treatments. The combination of hyperthermia and radiation has been shown to improve the initial tumour response, but local recurrence can still be a problem. Preoperative irradiation or cytoreductive surgery followed by radiation therapy is another strategy for the management of these tumours (McLeod and Thrall 1989).

Osteosarcoma, spindle cell sarcoma and poorly differentiated sarcoma

Osteosarcoma and a number of other sarcoma-type tumours, including spindle cell sarcomas and anaplastic sarcomas, also arise in the oral cavity. As a group, these represent up to 20% of canine malignant oral tumours. In gross appearance they may resemble fibrosarcoma, but in many cases they are more aggressive tumours. They present as a rapidly growing mass which may be friable or haemorrhagic and contain areas of necrosis (Fig. 15.8). These tumours frequently involve the bone and in the case of osteosarcoma the radiographic changes are similar to those occurring in the long bones, with a mixed pattern of osteolysis and production of an irregular bony matrix.

As with fibrosarcoma, these tumours are characterised by an infiltrative pattern of growth and they are often locally advanced by the time of diagnosis. A high proportion of these

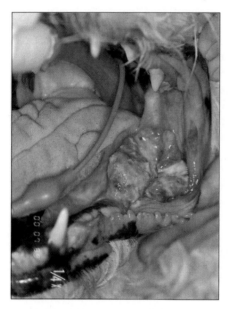

Fig. 15.8
Osteosarcoma in the caudal mandibular region.
The tumour is friable and contains areas of
necrosis.

tumours metastasize, usually via the haematogenous route to
the lungs and other internal organs.

The principles of management are essentially as for fibrosarcoma, although the prognosis is often worse due to the rapid
growth rate and higher risk of distant metastases. Small early
stage tumours may be surgically resected and cytoreductive
surgery combined with radiation therapy can be beneficial in
the management of more advanced tumours. Although most
soft tissue sarcomas are not very radioresponsive, the combination of radiation and hyperthermia has been shown to
improve the local control of these tumours.

MALIGNANT MELANOMA

Intraoral melanomas are the least common of the three major
types of canine oral neoplasm in our clinic. Oral melanoma
is rare in the cat.

In the dog, oral melanomas characteristically develop in
older animals, the mean age at onset is nine to 10 years. There
appears to be a sex predilection, with male dogs affected four
times more frequently than bitches. Certain breeds of dog,
particularly those with pigmented oral mucosa, eg, poodle

and pug, may be predisposed to this tumour. Common sites, in order of prevalence, are the gums (especially in the region of the molar teeth), the labial mucosa and the hard palate. The tumour usually presents as a rapidly growing friable and haemorrhagic soft tissue mass. The degree of pigmentation varies considerably, some tumours being heavily pigmented while others contain little to no pigment (Fig. 15.9). Secondary bacterial infection and necrosis may be present. Invasion of the bone is less common in oral melanoma than with SCC or fibrosarcoma and is reported to be in the order of 57% (Todoroff and Brodey 1979).

Canine oral melanomas are among the most malignant neoplasms encountered in companion animals. Local control can be achieved by wide surgical resections where the site of the tumour is appropriate or by radiation/hyperthermia. The human melanoma is generally regarded as being radioresistant, but our experience in the treatment of canine oral melanoma suggests these tumours are radiosensitive and when adjunctive hyperthermia is used, local response rates approaching 100% have been achieved. However, the major managemental problem presented by melanoma is the high incidence of both regional (nodal) and distant metastases. In the absence of an effective method for the prevention or treatment of disseminated melanoma, the prognosis for these tumours is poor and survival rates are in the order of three to six months.

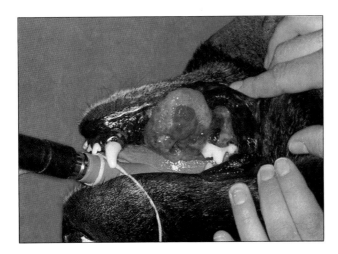

Fig. 15.9
Malignant melanoma of the mandible. This particular tumour has both pigmented and non-pigmented regions.

DIFFERENTIAL DIAGNOSIS OF ORAL TUMOURS

This article has discussed only the more common types of neoplasia occurring in the oral cavity. Other types of tumour, including mast cell tumours, plasmacytoma, salivary gland carcinoma and many more, occur sporadically in this site. Oral neoplasia must also be differentiated from a number of non-neoplastic conditions which affect the oral mucosa and lips, especially gingival hyperplasia, ulcerations related to viral infections (cats) or autoimmune conditions (eg, pemphigus group). Lingual/buccal granulomas occur in both cats and dogs in association with foreign bodies or anaerobic microorganisms. Calcinosis circumscripta can also occur in the tongue and soft tissues of the cheek in dogs. Histological examination of excised tissues may be necessary to differentiate between these conditions.

SUMMARY

The oral cavity and associated tissues are common sites for the development of tumours in cats and dogs. More than half the tumours occurring at this site are malignant, but the prognosis in such cases can often be improved by following a rational therapeutic approach. The key to the successful management of oral tumours can be summarized as follows:

(1)   Prompt detection, diagnosis and treatment of the tumour.
(2)   A representative biopsy of the tumour should be taken before definitive treatment. In many cases aggressive treatment may be indicated but cannot be justified without histological diagnosis.
(3)   An accurate assessment of the extent of the primary tumour with respect to adjacent tissues must be made before treatment and the treatment must be tailored to include all detected tumours with adequate margins.
(4)   Consideration must be given to the presence/absence of regional or distant metastases.

If these guidelines are followed the incidence of local tumour recurrence can be greatly reduced. The primary treatment is always more successful than subsequent treatments.

REFERENCES

Bostock, D. E. (1979) *Veterinary Pathology* **16**, 32.
Bostock, D. E. & White, R. A. S. (1987) *Journal of Comparative Pathology* **97**, 197.
Brodey, R. S. (1960) *American Journal of Veterinary Research* **21**, 787.
Dorn, C. R. & Priester, W. A. (1976) *Journal of the American Veterinary Medical Association* **169**, 1202.
Dubielzig, R. R., Goldschmidt, M. H. & Brodey, R. R. S. (1979) *Veterinary Pathology* **16**, 209.
Emms, S. & Harvey, C. E. (1986) *Journal of Small Animal Practice* **27**, 291.
Gillette, E. L., McChesney, S. L., Dewhirst, M. W. & Scott, R. J. (1987) *International Journal of Radiation Oncology, Biology & Physics* **13**, 1861.
Harvey, H. J. (1980) *Veterinary Clinics of North America* **10**, 821.
Harvey, H. J., MacEwan, E. G., Braun, D., Patnaik, A. K., Withrow, S. J. & Jongeward, S. (1981) *Journal of the American Veterinary Medical Association* **178**, 580.
Head, K. W. (1976) *Bulletin of the World Health Organization* **53**, 145.
Langham, R. R., Mostosky, V. V. & Schirmer, R. G. (1977) *Journal of the American Veterinary Medical Association* **170**, 820.
McLeod, D. & Thrall, D. E. (1989) *Veterinary Surgery* **18**, 1.
Salisbury, S. K. & Lantz, G. C. (1988) *Journal of the American Animal Hospital Association* **24**, 284.
Thompson, J. M., Gorman, N. T., Bleehen, N. M., Owen, L. N. & White, R. A. S. (1987) *Journal of Small Animal Practice* **28**, 457.
Thrall, D. E. (1984) *Journal of the American Medical Association* **84**, 826.
Thrall, D. E. & Dewhirst, M. W. (1986) *Contemporary Issues in Small Animal Practice*, Vol. 6, *Oncology* (ed. N. T. Gorman), Chapter 4. New York, Churchill Livingstone.
Todoroff, R. J. & Brodey, R. S. (1979) *Journal of the American Veterinary Medical Association* **175**, 567.
White, R. A. S., Jefferies, A. R. & Freedman, L. S. (1985a) *Journal of Small Animal Practice* **26**, 581.
White, R. A. S., Gorman, N. T., Watkins, S. B. & Brearley, M. J. (1985b) *Journal of Small Animal Practice* **26**, 693.
White, R. A. S., Jefferies, A. R. & Gorman, N. T. (1986) *Veterinary Record* **118**, 668.
White, R. A. S. (1987) *Veterinary Surgery* **16**, 105.
White, R. A. S. & Gorman, N. T. (1989) *Veterinary Surgery* **18**, 12.
Withrow, S. J. & Holmberg, D. L. (1983) *Journal of the American Animal Hospital Association* **19**, 273.

CHAPTER 16

Hormonal Alopecia in Dogs and Cats

KENNETH BAKER

INTRODUCTION

The dog or cat presented for examination with the complaint of hair loss is relatively common. Alopecia, however, may be a common feature of many dermatoses and it is therefore important that a thorough clinical examination be undertaken in each case.

Hair growth and replacement is a cyclical phenomenon initiated by the effect of increasing photoperiod on the hypothalamus, pineal, anterior pituitary and endocrine system. In some animals, eg, the rat, there is a definite wave pattern during moulting. However, in dogs, cats and man, hair is replaced mosaically: thus individual hairs in a compound follicle are replaced at different times. The cycle of hair growth is indicated diagrammatically in Fig. 16.1.

Plucking hair from the pelage will indicate the activity of the root. Telogen hairs have club-shaped roots which appear dull and dry when plucked, while the roots of actively growing hairs appear moist, stubby and thickened. In the compound follicles of the dog and cat, all the three stages may be present in the same follicle.

As alopecia may be caused by factors other than hormonal disturbances it is of value to examine with a microscope a

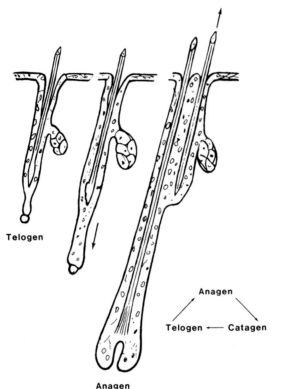

Fig. 16.1
Cycle of hair growth. Anagen—the active period of growth; catagen—the transition stage which follows anagen, growth of the hair ceases; telogen—the resting phase, the "germ" of the next hair below the club root of the old hair. The cycle will begin with active growth of the germ.

hair pluck to ascertain root stages. In hormonal alopecia, it will be easy to remove the hairs (epilation) and nearly all the roots will be in the telogen phase. The hair tips should be examined too. The tips of hairs which are exfoliating as a result of hormonal disturbance will be relatively normal, while in cases of hair loss associated with ectoparasitism the tips will be split and generally more ragged. Ectoparasitism is the major cause of alopecia and must always be eliminated before a diagnosis of hormonal alopecia is made. Hormonal alopecia predominantly affects middle-aged and older animals and characteristically it is not pruritic.

HYPOTHYROIDISM

Thyroidectomy prolongs the telogen phase while the adminis-tration of thyroxine shortens it; thus the thyroid gland is active in the initiation of normal hair growth and replacement. Hypothyroidism is probably the most commonly occurring hormonal alopecia in dogs, though there are no published statistics to support this. It can occur at any age, but most cases involve middle-aged or elderly animals. Nearly all cases of canine hypothyroidism are primary in origin, resulting from thyroid destruction. Commonly this is caused by lymphocytic thyroiditis with invasion of the thyroid tissue by lymphocytes, plasma cells and macrophages with destruc-tion of follicles. The majority of other cases are secondary and are due to pituitary neoplasms.

Initially hair loss is patchy (Fig. 16.2), the coat is dry, the hair is brittle and easily pulled out and the skin is cool to the touch. Hyperpigmentation develops: with time, the hair loss becomes extensive, with remnants remaining only on the head and extremities, and the skin becomes increasingly pigmented, wrinkled, thick and dry (Fig. 16.3). Secondary pyoderma and seborrhoeic dermatitis may occur. Fragmented skin tags may develop and the nails, like the hair, are brittle. The systemic signs are marked. Remaining hair is easily removed and nearly all hairs will be in the telogen phase, as indicated by the examination of hair plucks. The hypothyroidic skin is predisposed to bruising.

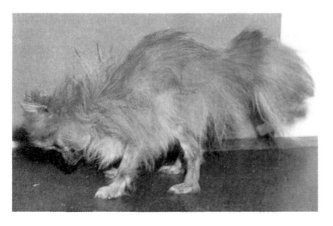

Fig. 16.2
Patchy alopecia caused by hypothyroidism in a pomeranian.

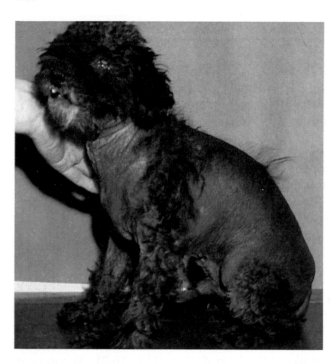

Fig. 16.3
Extensive alopecia in
a miniature poodle
with hypothyroidism.
The skin is puffy and
there is marked
hyperpigmentation.

DIAGNOSIS

A thorough clinical examination will reveal the accompanying systemic signs. Microscopic examination of a skin biopsy will show a thickened dermis in which there is evidence of collagen atrophy, follicular hyperkeratosis, follicular atrophy of the glandular adnexae and thinning of the epidermis. Increased dermal mucin is not always seen. Scott (1982) considers that with experience some endocrine dermatoses can be differentiated histopathologically.

There may be a normochromic, normocytic anaemia and serum cholesterol levels are usually much elevated. However, an abnormally high level of serum cholesterol is not specific for hypothyroidism.

Measurement of tri-iodothyronine (T3) and thyroxine (T4) levels alone, by radioimmune assay laboratories accustomed to human sera levels, is unsatisfactory when diagnosing hypothyroidism in dogs. Levels vary considerably in normal dogs according to breed, season and age and are much lower than those of man. Levels are affected by chronic illness and drug therapy, particularly with corticosteroids. However, Eckensall and Williams (1983) determined that the normal range for dogs of free T4 (7.5–50 pmol/litre) was comparable to the normal human range. Thus a free T4 kit may be used for estimating this fraction in dogs. As there is so much variation, consideration of levels of T4 alone should not be taken as an indication of thyroid activity: response to an injection of thyroid stimulating hormone will be of greater value. Free T4 estimations are made eight hours before and eight hours after the intravenous injection of 10 iu of thyrotrophic hormone. Little or no change in the T4 level between the two estimations is seen in cases of primary hypothyroidism, while in secondary hypothyroidism there is a marked elevation, approaching that of normal dogs after such stimulation. Commercial laboratories specializing in veterinary laboratory pathology are able to undertake these tests. Measurement of T4 levels may also be made using the enzyme-linked immunosorbent assay (ELISA) method.

The histopathological examination of thyroid biopsies is a valuable aid to diagnosis. Thyroid tissue should be submitted to the examining laboratory in 10% formalin. Usually in the early stages of primary hypothyroidism leucocyte infiltration and fibroplasia will not be seen. However, obvious atrophy is diagnosable. In secondary hypothyroidism the thyroid appears normal.

Only one report of spontaneous feline hypothyroidism, congenital in origin, has been recorded in the literature.

THERAPY

Thyroxine given at a dose rate of 20 μg/kg bodyweight orally twice daily usually leads to a satisfactory improvement but the animal should be clinically examined soon after therapy has commenced. A lower dose rate should be given where cardiac disease is present. While there is a dramatic systemic response, satisfactory hair growth may not be seen for several months, therefore dosage should be continued for at least 12 weeks before deciding on its effectiveness. Dose levels may then be diminished to the minimum effective level and maintained thereafter for life. Desiccated thyroid should not be used in the treatment of hypothyroidism because of its variable potency.

HYPERADRENOCORTICISM

Injudicious use of corticosteroid therapy may produce the clinical signs of hyperadrenocorticism. Corticosteroid therapy should never be used to control pruritus until the possibility of ectoparasitic infestation has been eliminated. It is not unusual for the referral case to be one of ectoparasitism which has been treated for many months with corticosteroids; iatrogenic Cushing's disease may be the result.

Natural causes of hyperadrenocorticism in the dog are idiopathic adrenal hyperplasia, adrenal cortical tumour and pituitary tumour. These conditions primarily occur in middle-aged or older dogs of either sex. As with hypothyroidism, marked systemic clinical signs are seen. These may be varied. Characteristically there is polydipsia,polyuria, polyphagia, lethargy, weakness and hepatomegaly with enlargement of the abdomen, which is pendulous and lacks tone. Muscle wastage is apparent. A patchy alopecia of the trunk develops, often with complete hairlessness of the trunk: the head and extremities are usually spared (Fig. 16.4). The skin feels thin, dry and scaly, is wrinkled and inelastic: it is easily damaged and healing is delayed. A pinched skin fold shows slow recoil. Comedomes (blackheads) are noticeable on the ventral chest and inguinal region and the testicles are small and soft. Calcinosis cutis (not specific) may be seen. Blood vessels appear unusually prominent through the atrophied wrinkled skin. Hyperpigmentation is variable and is not as evident compared with the skin in hypothyroidism. Petechiae and ecchymoses are evident. There may be large spots (macules), each with a scaly periphery on the trunk. As with hypothyroidism, there may be secondary pyoderma or seborrhoea, or both.

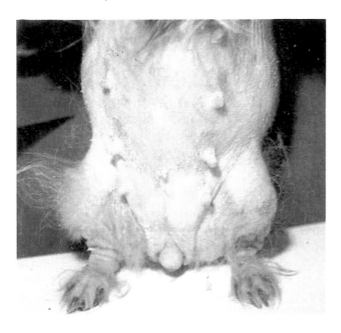

Fig. 16.4
A case of
hyperadrenocorticism
in the dog, with
enlarged abdomen
and seborrhoea.

DIAGNOSIS

With hyperadrenocorticism there are marked haematological changes: neutrophilia, lymphopenia and eosinopenia, as shown by a differential white cell count and an absolute eosinophil count. Certain serum enzyme levels are often raised, for example, serum alanine aminotransferase and serum alkaline phosphatase: serum cholesterol may also be raised. The specific gravity of the urine is reduced to 1.006–1.010. Radiographically there is osteoporosis and evidence of soft tissue calcification.

Plasma and blood cortisol levels are elevated but several samples should be examined. Because of the possible variation in cortisol levels at different times of day, samples should be taken at the same time each day, using lithium heparin tubes, and estimations made using the radioimmunoassay method for greatest accuracy.

Confirmation may be made by the adrenocorticotrophic hormone stimulation test. A pre-test sample of blood is collected in heparin after overnight starvation, 60 minutes before the intramuscular or intravenous injection of 0.25 mg of adrenocorticotrophic hormone (Synachthen; Ciba): a further blood sample is collected one hour later. In cortical hyperplasia there is usually marked increase in the plasma cortisol level. However, there is little or no increase of the plasma cortisol level in adrenal cortical neoplasia.

Recent research has indicated that the adrenocorticotrophic hormone stimulation test does not always distinguish between hyperadrenocorticism caused by adrenocortical tumours and that caused by pituitary dysfunction. The dexamethasone suppression test is more accurate for this purpose and may be used to distinguish between adrenal cortical hyperplasia and adrenal cortical neoplasia. The dog is starved overnight and a heparinized blood sample is taken. Twelve hours later 0.1 mg/kg bodyweight of dexamethasone is given by mouth and a further sample taken the following morning. In dogs with adrenal cortical hyperplasia the plasma cortisol levels show a decrease of less than 50%, while in dogs with adrenal cortical neoplasia little or no decrease is evident.

Practitioners should ascertain from their examining laboratories the special requirements for the collection of plasma samples and their transport before submitting them.

TREATMENT

There are two approaches to therapy in dogs, medical and surgical. Of these, the former is to be preferred. Mitotane (Lysodren; Bristol-Myers) is selectively cytotoxic for the adrenal cortex. It is given at a dose rate of 50 mg/kg bodyweight by mouth daily (divided dose rate) for one week, during which time the clinical signs are assessed, reducing the dose rate if necessary and administering hydrocortisone orally daily at a dose rate of 1.5 mg/kg bodyweight commencing on day 3 and terminating on day 7. Maintenance dosage of mitotane is 50 mg/kg bodyweight weekly thereafter, monitoring the systemic response and giving additional hydrocortisone if necessary. Alternatively mitotane may be given daily in dose rates sufficient to produce the desired clinical response and then a once weekly dose of 50 mg/kg bodyweight is given.

Cortisol producing neoplasms of the adrenal cortex occur in one in 10 cases of hyperadrenocorticism. They should be removed by unilateral adrenalectomy. As the remaining adrenal cortex will be atrophied, replacement therapy will be essential; prednisolone may be given on alternate days with clinical assessment at regular intervals.

Where there is bilateral hyperplasia of the adrenal cortex, both adrenal glands are removed. Subsequently very careful management for hypo-adrenocorticism will be necessary.

Surgical removal of pituitary neoplasms associated with hyperadrenocorticism poses numerous obvious difficulties for both the surgeon and clinician. It should not be considered unless the owner has been told of the difficulties and the subsequent problems of clinical management for the remainder of the dog's life.

Feline hyperadrenocorticism does occur although no reports of therapy in the literature have been seen by the author.

PITUITARY DWARFISM

Pituitary dwarfism is a rare disease but has been reported from a number of countries. It may be transmitted by an autosomal recessive gene. Most cases have been recorded in German shepherd dogs. Affected animals are normal for the first few months of life, but then failure of the pituitary body to produce adequate growth hormone results in dwarfism and bilateral alopecia. Characteristically affected dogs are of normal proportions but of small stature, with marked retention of the secondary (lanugo) hair with failure to produce the adult primary hair (top coat). The coat is soft and fluffy (undercoat). Temperament may be variable from persistent aggression and nervousness to apparent normality. The external genitalia may or may not be juvenile in form and patchy or generalized hyperpigmentation of the skin may be seen. Radiologically the skeletal bone plates appear to be arrested in development with skeletal agenesis. The condition will not be noticeable until four months of age.

Therapy is undesirable. Normally behaved dogs can lead active lives while others should be destroyed. Parents of the affected dog should not be mated together again.

GROWTH HORMONE RESPONSIVE ALOPECIA

Though reported in North America (Parker and Scott 1980) in several breeds (chow, keeshond, pomeranian and miniature poodle), growth hormone responsive alopecia has not been reported in the British Isles. Affected dogs are normal initially, with the disease beginning in the second and third year of life. Extensive bilateral symmetrical alopecia with hyperpigmentation is reported, with no systemic signs. Decreased dermal elastin is suggestive, with epidermal and follicular hyperkeratosis, associated follicular dilation, hyperpigmentation and sebaceous gland atrophy; thinning of the dermis occurs. However, these are also seen in hypothyroidism. Normal hair growth can be restored with growth hormone therapy.

The diagnosis must be based on the history, clinical signs, dermal histopathology and response to growth hormone therapy (5–10 units of pig growth hormone is given subcutaneously on alternate days).

SERTOLI CELL TUMOUR

Sertoli cell tumour most commonly occurs in the cryptorchid testicle but not all such tumours will be associated with feminization and alopecia. As with hyperadrenocorticism and hypothyroidism, there are marked systemic changes which assist diagnosis. Alopecia develops in the inguinal and flank areas. These become confluent and there may be extensive loss of hair. The skin, though bald in affected areas, is often normal in appearance; seborrhoea may be seen. Bilateral hyperpigmentation occurs as the disease develops.

Histopathologically, the glandular adnexae are small and there is follicular hyperkeratosis. The degenerative changes of the epidermis and dermis of hyperadrenocorticism and hypothyroidism are not seen. Behavioural changes are apparent. There is lethargy, lack of libido and the animal becomes sexually attractive to other males. Gynaecomastia is seen. The prepuce appears larger, and is soft and pendulous. Affected dogs may adopt a feminine urination posture. Usually the tumour is found in a cryptorchid testicle but not invariably so. Neoplastic scrotal testicles usually are palpably large and firm. The non-neoplastic scrotal testicle feels small and soft.

Although the clinical signs are characteristic, the diagnosis should exclude the feminizing syndrome of male dogs unassociated with Sertoli cell tumour. The clinical examination should include palpation of the abdomen and radiography of the thorax because of the possibility of metastasis. Anaemia, a result of bone marrow depression, may occur in oestrogen secreting Sertoli cell tumours.

Removal of the neoplastic testicle is essential and will result in a dramatic clinical response, though hair growth may not be apparent for several months. Regular shampoos for secondary seborrhoea may be considered desirable.

MALE FEMINIZING SYNDROME

Male feminizing syndrome is a less common disorder than Sertoli cell tumour which is not associated with testicular neoplasia. The aetiology is not known. Abnormal levels of oestrogen and testosterone were not detected in five affected animals examined by Matthews and Comhaire (1975), who hypothesized that a circulatory anti-androgen is responsible for the clinical signs.

The clinical signs resemble those of dogs with functional Sertoli cell tumours (Fig. 16.5) and similarly there may be seborrhoea and pruritus with hyperpigmentation and hyperkeratosis. Castration will restore the normal hair growth. Regular mild skin baths should be given to control the seborrhoea. A testosterone implant (1 mg/lb bodyweight) is effective also.

The disease should be distinguished from other conditions in which seborrhoea occurs, and from functional Sertoli cell tumour.

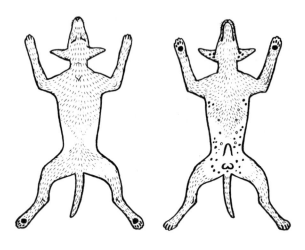

Fig. 16.5
Diagram of alopecic areas in
male feminizing syndrome in
the dog.

PROGESTERONE-INDUCED ALOPECIA

A small percentage of bitches in late pregnancy and lactation
develop a diffuse alopecia of the trunk without obvious skin
lesions, hyperpigmentation or pruritus (Fig. 16.6). The bitch
appears normal but the hair is easily depilated.

The condition can be reproduced experimentally by oral
dosing with progesterone to adult normal bitches. In the
naturally occurring case, no therapy is desirable or required.
Hair replacement will commence upon weaning. As progestogens are now widely used in veterinary practice the possibility
of iatrogenic alopecia should be considered.

FEMALE HYPEROESTROGENISM (OVARIAN IMBALANCE TYPE 1)

Female hyperoestrogenism is an uncommon dermatosis which
may be produced by ovarian imbalance or by prolonged
oestrogen therapy. The condition has been little researched.
It is probably not a simple problem of hyperoestrogenism.

In affected animals the oestrous cycle is irregular: there
may be gynaecomastia and vulval enlargement, and the
perineum and vulval area is characteristically deeply pigmented, with dusky hyperpigmentation in the alopecic areas

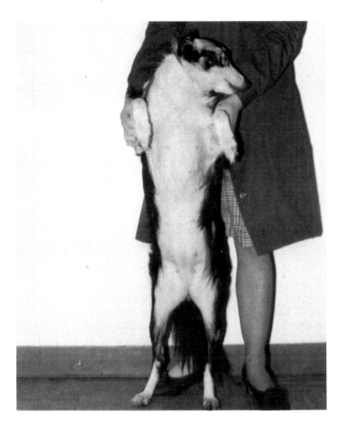

Fig. 16.6
Progesterone-induced
alopecia in a five-
year old collie bitch.

in advanced cases. Loss of hair commences in the inguinal region and extends to the ventral abdomen and flanks, affected areas being completely denuded (Figs 16.7 and 16.8). There may be seborrhoea oleosa and pruritus. Comedomes are observed in the posterior ventral abdomen. As in other causes of seborrhoea a ceruminous otitis is often present.

The possibility of hypothyroidism or hyperadrenocorticism should be determined by the appropriate tests. Therapy of choice is ovariohysterectomy. Hair replacement will be complete in six months and the hyperpigmentation will gradually disappear.

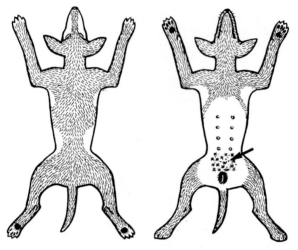

Fig. 16.7
Diagram of alopecic areas in hyperoestrogenism in the bitch. Note vulval hypertrophy and hyperpigmentation, gynaecomastia and comedomes (arrowed).

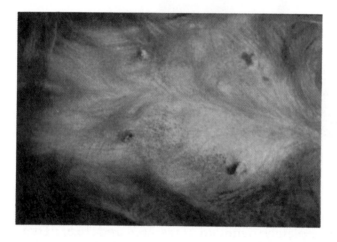

Fig. 16.8
A case of hyperoestrogenism in the bitch, with gynaecomastia, ventral alopecia and comedome formation.

FEMALE HYPOOESTROGENISM (OVARIAN IMBALANCE TYPE 2)

A consequence of juvenile ovariohysterectomy may be urinary incontinence with infantile nipples and vulva; quite rarely an extensive alopecia of the ventral abdomen, thorax and flank may develop (Fig. 16.9) which is more extensive than so-called female hyperoestrogenism and hyperpigmentation. Comedome formation and seborrhoea are not associated with it.

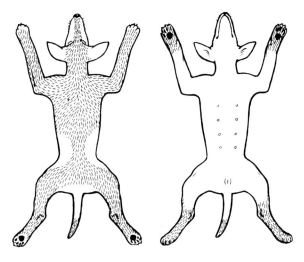

Fig. 16.9
Diagram of alopecic areas in hypooestrogenism in the bitch. Note juvenile vulva and nipples.

There is a good response to oestradiol therapy. A daily dose rate of up to 1 mg is given for four weeks. Dosage is then resumed for a further three weeks after a break of one week. This cycle should be repeated, after which hair growth should be apparent. Thereafter a weekly dose of up to 1 mg may be necessary, with adjustment. When prescribing oestrogen therapy for long periods consider the potential danger of bone marrow depression.

FELINE HORMONAL ALOPECIA

Feline hormonal alopecia (Fig. 16.10), which is of unknown aetiology, occurs relatively commonly in neutered and entire males and females of middle age.

Unlike hyperadrenocorticism and hypothyroidism, the skin is apparently normal. Sections reveal no abnormality other than a great reduction in the number of primary follicles with the remainder and the secondary hairs in the resting phase. In the advanced case, there is bilaterally symmetrical alopecia. In some cases hair is only retained on the head (Fig. 16.11). However, the skin does not become bald for there is some retention of the secondary follicles. In this the hair coat has a similarity to the normal prepubertal pelage and

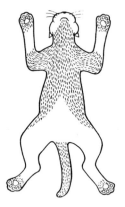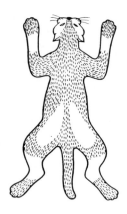

Fig. 16.10
Diagram of alopecic areas in symmetrical feline hormonal alopecia.

may therefore indicate some interference with the normal effect of the sex hormone on hair follicles.

Ectoparasitic causes of alopecia in the cat are accompanied by self-excoriation, with obvious skin lesions, and the hair is broken and shows lick marks. No abnormal levels of plasma cortisol, thyroxine, androgens or oestrogens have been reported in affected cats. Implantation of affected cats with 25 mg testosterone will often produce satisfactory hair growth, though it may need to be repeated at six-month intervals. Undesirable male characteristics may develop also and therefore it may be used in conjunction with oestrogen intramuscularly.

Progestogens such as megestrol acetate (Ovarid; Pitman-Moore) are used also, at a dose of 5 mg megestrol daily by mouth diminishing as hair growth occurs. Thereafter, maintenance may be necessary, with 5 mg weekly. Owners may report that treated cats have developed a more placid temperament with a tendency to weight gain. Synthetic thyroxine has also been used: a dose of 0.3 mg sodium levothyroxine is given daily for three months followed by 0.3 mg twice weekly.

DIABETES MELLITUS

Alopecia is commonly associated with diabetes mellitus in man but the author has not seen this in affected dogs or cats.

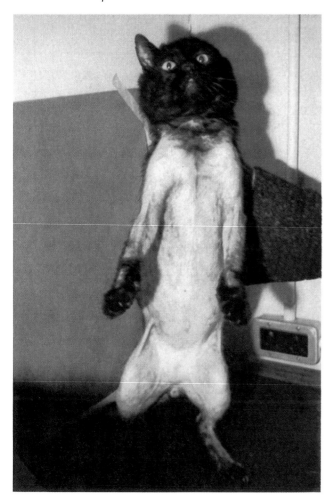

Fig. 16.11
Extensive hair loss in
a five-year-old
neutered male cat
suffering from feline
hormonal alopecia.

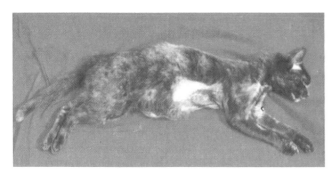

Fig. 16.12
Biliary carcinoma
associated with
patchy alopecia in a
cat.

In an extensive survey of dogs with diabetes mellitus in the United Kingdom, Foster (1975) reported that 7% of cases had skin lesions but these were not specified.

It should be noted that severe liver disease may produce marked skin pathology; an early presenting symptom may be diffuse hair loss. This may be associated with the failure of the liver to control hormone levels.

ACANTHOSIS NIGRICANS

Though acanthosis nigricans is often considered to be caused by an endocrine alopecia, there is no evidence to support this. The term should be reserved for a disease of man associated with gastric adenocarcinoma. In dogs, acanthosis of skin folds in the axillary and inguinal region may be secondary to a variety of non-specific dermatoses.

REFERENCES

Erkensall, P. D. & Williams, M. E. (1983) *Journal of Small Animal Practice* **24**, 525.
Foster, S. J. (1975) *Journal of Small Animal Practice* **16**, 295.
Matthews, D. & Comhaire, F. (1975) *British Veterinary Journal* **131**, 65.
Parker, W. M. & Scott, D. W. (1980) *Journal of the American Animal Hospital Association* **16**, 824.
Scott, D. W. (1982) *Journal of the American Animal Hospital Association* **18**, 173.

CHAPTER 17

Diabetes Mellitus

ELSPETH MILNE

INTRODUCTION

Diabetes mellitus is a relatively common endocrine disorder in dogs and cats, associated with a relative or absolute lack of insulin from the pancreas and characterized by glucose intolerance. Successful management requires a long term commitment on the part of the owners and their veterinary surgeon to monitoring and treating the case, and a thorough understanding of the aetiology so that appropriate therapy can be given.

NORMAL ENDOCRINE PANCREAS (Fig. 17.1)

The pancreas is a mixed endocrine and exocrine gland. The endocrine secretion is produced by cells arranged in clusters known as islets of Langerhans. The islets are interspersed among the acini of the exocrine pancreas and consist of two main cell types, the alpha and beta cells, which produce the hormones glucagon and insulin, respectively. These hormones are directly involved in the maintenance of blood glucose levels but also have effects on lipid and protein metabolism.

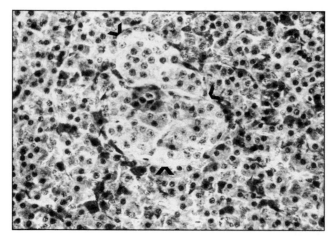

Fig. 17.1
Normal pancreas
showing islet of
Langerhans
(delineated by
arrows) amongst the
acini of the exocrine
pancreas.

By their opposing action, blood insulin and glucagon maintain blood glucose levels within critical limits in the normal animal (Table 17.1). Several hormones produced by other endocrine glands including progesterone, growth hormone and glucocorticoids also oppose the action of insulin on blood glucose and are very important in the aetiology of the disease.

Table 17.1 Effects of insulin and glucagon.

Insulin	Secreted in response to hyperglycaemia.
	Facilitates uptake of glucose, amino acids, fatty acids and potassium from the blood therefore *decreases* blood glucose.
	Inhibits glucose production by gluconeogenesis and glycogenolysis.
	Inhibits catabolism of lipid and protein.
	Inhibits ketone production.
Glucagon	Secreted in response to hypoglycaemia.
	Opposes the above actions of insulin, therefore *increases* blood glucose.

AETIOLOGY (Table 17.2)

Diabetes mellitus is caused by an absolute or relative lack of insulin which results in impairment of uptake of glucose by peripheral tissues. The body attempts to increase the supply of glucose to the tissues by stimulating gluconeogenesis and glycogenolysis, oxidation of fats and protein catabolism. Ketones are produced during oxidation of fats. The overall effect is therefore an increase in glucose production, and a decrease in its utilization leading to hyperglycaemia. When the renal threshold for glucose is exceeded, glycosuria will occur which causes osmotic diuresis, polyuria and polydipsia. Ketonuria may also be present. The cause of the relative or absolute lack of insulin differs between the species.

AETIOLOGY IN THE DOG

Secondary diabetes mellitus associated with hormone antagonism or obesity appears to be the most common form in the dog. High levels of circulating progesterone, eg, in pregnancy, dioestrus or during therapy with certain progestogens (eg, medroxyprogesterone acetate) stimulate growth hormone production, the latter being a strong antagonist to insulin. Similarly when glucocorticoid levels are high either in

Table 17.2

Primary diabetes mellitus

    Congenital hypoplasia of islets.
    Senile atrophy of islets.

Secondary diabetes mellitus

    Following pancreatitis.
    Excessive secretion of hormones antagonistic to insulin,
      ie, *progesterone, growth hormone, glucocorticoids,*
      oestrogen, androgens catecholamines or thyroxine.
    Excessive administration of hormones, ie, long-term
      progestogen or glucocorticoid therapy
    Obesity
    Immune-mediated insulin resistance?

hyperadrenocorticalism or after administration, insulin antagonism will occur, which in some cases can precipitate frank diabetes mellitus. Obesity also alters blood glucose homeostasis to create insulin resistance. The role of immune-mediated insulin resistance in canine diabetes mellitus is at present uncertain.

In the initial stages of insulin antagonism, blood insulin levels will be high in an attempt to compensate. At this stage the diabetic state may not be permanent but if the cause of antagonism is not removed, beta cell exhaustion and permanent diabetes mellitus will occur.

AETIOLOGY IN THE CAT

The aetiology of diabetes mellitus is less well understood in cats. Deposition of the protein amyloid is a frequent finding in the beta cells of diabetic and some normal cats. This is associated with glucose intolerance, but its exact role in the disease is uncertain. Other factors which have been associated with diabetes mellitus in cats are hyperadrenocorticalism, pituitary tumours, obesity and megoestrol acetate therapy. Unlike entire bitches, entire queens are apparently not predisposed to diabetes. Stress glycosuria is very common in cats with a variety of illnesses. It is usually transient but if prolonged, or beta cell dysfunction is present, it may precipitate a permanent diabetic state.

HISTORY

The major features of the history are polyuria and polydipsia, usually together with polyphagia and weight loss. These may be of gradual or sudden onset. Bitches may have a history of recent oestrus and may have shown transient polydipsia at previous oestrus periods. Both dogs and cats may have received recent progestogen or glucocorticoid therapy.

Table 17.3 Incidence of diabetes mellitus.

	Canine	Feline
Incidence in population	1:200	1:800
Sex incidence before puberty	50% F 50% M	50% F 50% M
Sex incidence after puberty	65% entire F 17% spayed F 17% M (entire or castrated)	50% F (entire or spayed) 50% M (entire or castrated)
Age incidence	Usually middle aged to old, peak incidence 7–9 years	
Breeds	Common in small breeds especially dachshunds, poodles and terriers. Rarer in larger breeds but samoyeds and rottweilers predisposed?	Siamese predisposed?

M Male   F Female

CLINICAL SIGNS

Uncomplicated cases present with polyuria, polydipsia, polyphagia, weight loss, mild dehydration and, in 50% of cases, hepatomegaly caused by a fatty liver. Despite weight loss, many animals are still obese at presentation. In dogs, unilateral or bilateral cataracts may be present although in this age group, some may be senile rather than diabetic cataracts. Diabetic cataracts are very rare in cats. Most uncomplicated cases are bright or only slightly depressed when presented. If ketoacidosis is present, there may be severe depression or coma, anorexia, vomiting, a ketotic breath and oliguria rather than polyuria. Ketoacidotic cats may be jaundiced.

DIFFERENTIAL DIAGNOSIS (Table 17.4)

It is beyond the scope of this article to discuss the differential diagnosis in detail but it should be borne in mind that hyperadrenocorticalism and stress glycosuria may precipitate the diabetic state and that hyperadrenocorticalism and diabetes mellitus may exist concurrently. Mild hyperglycaemia and glycosuria may sometimes occur in hyperadrenocorticalism, hepatic failure or stress glycosuria whereas in the Fanconi syndrome, a rare disorder in which there is a failure of the renal tubules to reabsorb glucose, glycosuria will be present without hyperglycaemia.

DIAGNOSIS

The history and clinical signs of polyuria, polydipsia, polyphagia and weight loss are not pathognomonic of diabetes mellitus and laboratory confirmation is required in all cases.

SPECIFIC TESTS

Fasting blood glucose levels consistently exceeding 8.5 mmol/litre (normal values 3–5 mmol/litre). These must be taken on two or more occasions at least eight hours after the last meal. This is best measured by a laboratory but Glucostix (Ames) can be useful, especially if the result is measured using an instrument such as the Glucometer (Ames) (Fig. 17.2).

Urine analysis. Glycosuria is present indicating that the blood glucose level has exceeded the renal threshold of 8–11 mmol/litre. Ketonuria is often present initially. Both can be detected using Keto-Diastix (Ames).

Table 17.4 Differential diagnosis of diabetes mellitus.

Renal disease
Hyperadrenocorticalism
Pyometra
Diabetes insipidus
Psychogenic polydipsia
Hepatic failure
Stress glycosuria
Fanconi syndrome

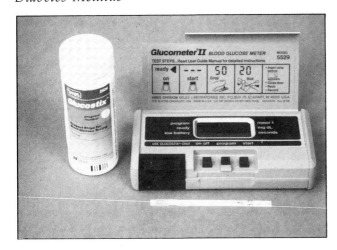

Fig. 17.2
Ames Glucostix and
Glucometer for rapid
blood glucose
assays.

Glucose tolerance test. This may be necessary in cases where the diagnosis is uncertain. It is not advisable, or necessary, if there is marked hyperglycaemia.

Oral or intravenous glucose tolerance tests (IVGTT) can be done but the latter is more reliable as it is not influenced by the motility and absorptive capacity of the gut. The IVGTT is simply performed (Table 17.5 and Fig. 17.3). In normal animals, the blood glucose has returned to half the immediate post-injection level in 20 min and is back to normal within an hour. If glucose intolerance is present, return to the basal level is delayed.

Table 17.5 Protocol for the IVGTT in dogs and cats.

(1) Starve animal overnight
(2) Take basal blood glucose sample before test
(3) Give 1g glucose/kg bodyweight as a 50% solution intravenously over 30 s
(4) Take further blood glucose samples immediately after glucose administration then at 10, 15, 20 and 40 min. Collect the samples from a different vein from the one used for glucose administration

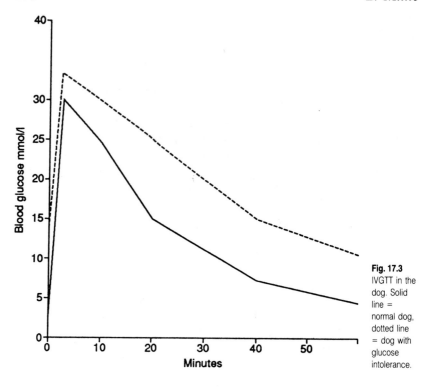

Fig. 17.3
IVGTT in the dog. Solid line = normal dog, dotted line = dog with glucose intolerance.

NON-SPECIFIC TESTS

Liver enzymes. Serum alkaline phosphatase (SAP), gamma glutamyl transpeptidase (GGT) and to a lesser extent alanine aminotransferase (ALT) may be raised because of a fatty liver. Alkaline phosphatase is less reliable in cats because of its short half-life in this species.

Serum lipids. The serum may be visibly lipaemic and serum triglycerides and cholesterol may be elevated due to disturbances of fat metabolism.

Blood urea. May be increased up to approximately 20 mmol/litre because of dehydration and protein catabolism. High levels following rehydration suggest concurrent renal disease.

Serum electrolytes. Na^+, K^+, HCO_3^- and blood pH may be low, especially in ketoacidosis.

TREATMENT

Before long-term treatment is contemplated, the implications should be explained to the owner, as daily insulin injections and urine glucose testing will be required for the rest of the animal's life in most cases. The cost of laboratory tests and hospitalization during stabilization may sometimes be prohibitive although insulin itself is not very expensive. If the owner is unwilling to accept the treatment regime immediate euthanasia of the animal is advisable.

TREATMENT OF DIABETIC KETOACIDOSIS

Cases with ketonuria but no signs of ketoacidosis can be treated as uncomplicated cases but if signs of ketoacidosis are present, particularly ketoacidotic coma, emergency treatment is required. This involves correction of fluid deficit, acid–base balance and electrolyte disturbances and reduction of blood glucose and ketone levels.

Correction of fluid deficit

Assess dehydration by clinical examination and, if possible, also by PCV and total protein estimations. Fluid loss is usually 10–20% bodyweight in ketoacidosis, eg, a 15 kg dog which is 10% dehydrated will have a fluid deficit of 1.5 litres. Give intravenous fluids at a rate of 20–40 ml/kg/hour for the first 2 h then decrease the rate so half of the deficit is restored by 12 h. Over the next 36 h give the remainder of the deficit plus the daily maintenance requirement of 40 ml/kg/day.

Correction of acid–base balance

Ideally, blood pH and bicarbonate deficit should be measured but since this is rarely available, lactated Ringer's solution (or Hartmann's solution) is the fluid of choice. It must be assumed that a significant bicarbonate deficit is present which can be corrected by adding 4 mM sodium bicarbonate/kg bodyweight to the lactated Ringer's solution (0.34 g NaHCO$_3$/kg body weight). This should be added *evenly* to the lactated Ringer's solution required. Alkalinizing solutions should never be given as a bolus. If in doubt about adding bicarbonate, lactated Ringer's solution should be used alone.

Correction of electrolyte disturbances

Serum sodium and potassium may be low, and potassium will fall further when insulin therapy is commenced, because insulin stimulates uptake of potassium into tissues. If serum electrolytes cannot be monitored frequently, it is much safer to give oral rather than intravenous potassium supplementation for the first few days.

Reduction of blood glucose and ketone levels

Dehydration will result in inadequate absorption of insulin given subcutaneously or intramuscularly so these routes cannot be used in ketoacidosis. Soluble insulin (see Table 17.6) must therefore be used to correct ketoacidosis as it is the only form suitable for intravenous use.

Table 17.6 Types of insulin available.

Insulin	Peak activity* (h)	Duration* (h)	Route of administration
Short-acting (soluble, regular or crystalline)	½–6	1–10	iv, im or sc
Intermediate-acting (isophane or insulin zinc suspension)	4–12	8–24	sc
Long-acting (protamine zinc insulin)	5–14	8–30	sc

*The figures given are for dogs and are usually lower in cats, which metabolize insulin more rapidly.
iv intravenous, im intramuscular, sc subcutaneous

It is easiest to give the insulin as repeated intravenous boluses at the following empirical rates:

Large dogs   1 unit of insulin/kg bodyweight
Small dogs   2 units/kg
Cats   0.5 unit/kg

The bolus should be repeated every 2 h until blood glucose (which should also be measured two-hourly), falls to half the original level (in most cases the original level will be 20–30 mmol/litre). The animal can then be treated as an uncomplicated case.

TREATMENT OF UNCOMPLICATED DIABETES MELLITUS

Treatment of precipitating factors

The possibility that the diabetic state has been precipitated secondarily, eg, by high progesterone or glucocorticoid levels (either exogenous or endogenous) should be considered and steps taken to correct such factors. If the cause of secondary diabetes mellitus is removed before beta cell exhaustion occurs, the state may be reversible. Entire bitches should be spayed once blood glucose is under control, although it has been suggested that oestrus can be suppressed using proligestone (Delvosteron; Gistbrocades) which does not stimulate growth hormone production (Evans and Sutton 1988). Its use for this purpose in clinical cases has not been fully evaluated.

Oral hypoglycaemic therapy

This is of little value as nearly all diabetics are already insulin dependent when first presented. Metformin (Glucophage; Lipha) has been used in dogs at 250–500 mg twice daily with food but only in rare cases of mild glucose intolerance associated with obesity, or in combination with insulin therapy to decrease the dose of insulin required. Glucophage is not licensed for veterinary use.

Stabilization on insulin

Stabilization is easier if the animal is hospitalized, but it can sometimes be achieved at home. It is more practicable to stabilize the animal on the basis of its urine glucose rather than blood glucose although it is helpful to monitor both during stabilization. A urine sample should be collected first thing in the morning and tested for glucose and ketones using, eg, KetoDiastix (Ames). The result is interpreted as shown in Table 17.7.

It is safer to give the insulin during or immediately after the morning meal to avoid the risk of hypoglycaemia if the food is not eaten. If the animal refuses the food, only half the insulin should be given that day. Cats metabolize insulin more quickly than dogs and some may require an intermediate-acting insulin every 12 h or a long-acting insulin once daily (see section on investigation of instability).

Diet

Divide the daily food requirement into a small morning meal and a larger afternoon meal. It is very important to keep the diet exactly the same at all times and titbits must be avoided. Proprietary diets such as Hill's Canine or Feline r/d are suitable, although diets can be made up using a ratio of carbohydrate to protein of approximately 1:4. The addition of

Table 17.7 Interpretation of glucose test.

0% glucose	Give 2 units of insulin less than the previous day as overnight blood glucose is below the renal threshold and could be very low.
0.1–0.5% glucose	This is the ideal level. Keep the insulin dose the same as the previous day.
1–2% glucose	Increase the insulin dose by 2 units in dogs or 1 unit in cats which are more insulin-sensitive.

Start insulin therapy with an intermediate-acting insulin given once-daily by subcutaneous injection.
Suitable starting doses are as follows:
Dog >10 kg—4 units; dog <10 kg—2 units; cat—1 unit.

some soluble but unabsorbable carbohydrate such as guar gum helps to delay absorption of glucose and decrease insulin requirements in human diabetics and may have some value in small animals. Free access to water is allowed. If ketonuria is present initially, 1 teaspoon of sodium bicarbonate powder can be added per 500 ml of drinking water for the first few days.

Daily routine

The following is a suggested daily management routine:

08.00   Collect and test urine
08.30   Give $\frac{1}{4}$ to $\frac{1}{3}$ of daily food
08.35   Inject insulin if animal has eaten
16.00   Give remaining $\frac{3}{4}$ to $\frac{2}{3}$ of daily food

The afternoon feed is timed so that the post prandial blood glucose level reaches its peak *before* the blood insulin activity has peaked (approximately 10 h after injection), ie, blood glucose is peaking at a time when blood insulin is increasing uptake of glucose at a maximal rate.

TREATMENT OF ACUTE HYPOGLYCAEMIA

Acute hypoglycaemia generally follows insulin overdosage, administration of insulin to an animal which has not eaten or excessive exercise. Signs vary from nervousness, muscle twitching and lethargy to coma or convulsions. The owner should be advised on emergency treatment, ie, if the animal is conscious, feed a meal containing glucose powder or if unconscious, carefully smear syrup on the tongue. If an episode occurs in the surgery give 2–10 ml of 50% glucose by slow intravenous injection.

DISCHARGING THE DIABETIC

Once the animal's thirst is under control and approximately the same dose of insulin has been required for several consecutive days, it can be discharged. An instruction sheet explaining all aspects of the management including signs and treatment of hypoglycaemia should be given to the owner. It is helpful in the event of instability for the owner to have kept a record of daily urine glucose and ketone levels, insulin dose, food eaten and weekly bodyweight. The owner should practise the urine dipstick test and give a subcutaneous injection before leaving the surgery. Approximately 45 min need to be set aside to discuss the instruction sheet and to practise injection and urine testing techniques.

Exercise should be kept to a minimum initially as the dog will have been stabilized for little exercise when hospitalized and hypoglycaemia may occur if exercise is suddenly increased. Urine dipsticks, insulin and disposable insulin syringes should be supplied. Routine health checks are required after one week then at three-monthly intervals.

INVESTIGATION OF INSTABILITY

The patient is poorly stabilized if:

(1)   Clinical signs are not controlled
(2)   Persistent morning glycosuria is present
(3)   Signs of hypoglycaemia occur

Most causes of instability are simply resolved. These include irregular inappropriate feeding (especially of titbits), inability to administer insulin properly, inadequate or too vigorous mixing of insulin, out-of-date or wrongly stored insulin or urine dipsticks and incorrect interpretation of urine dipsticks. If these simple causes can be eliminated but instability persists, serial blood glucose samples should be taken every 4 h for 24 h to produce a graph of blood glucose throughout the day. It is most practicable to hospitalize the animal for this, trying to follow the owner's regime as closely as possible.

INSULIN RESISTANCE

Insulin resistance is the most common of the more complex causes of instability and is suspected when increasing doses of insulin are required. It is diagnosed by demonstrating a persistent hyperglycaemia throughout 24 h, despite high doses of insulin. It is likely to be due to insulin antagonism, eg, during dioestrus or pregnancy, and possible initiating causes should be explored and treated. The role of antibody formation against exogenous insulin is uncertain but changing from a bovine insulin to porcine insulin is sometimes beneficial if no other cause can be found for the resistance. Porcine insulin is identical in primary structure to canine insulin and is likely to be less antigenic.

INSULIN-INDUCED HYPERGLYCAEMIA

Consistently high urine glucose levels in the morning can sometimes be caused by *excessive* insulin administration. A large dose initially causes a sudden fall in blood glucose to subnormal levels. This stimulates the sudden release of antagonistic hormones which quickly increase blood glucose again causing an overswing towards hyperglycaemia. Heavy glycosuria will be present the following day and the owner will feel obliged to increase the insulin dose still further. In these cases the insulin dose should be halved and the animal restabilized.

RAPID METABOLISM OF INSULIN

Some dogs, but particularly cats, metabolize exogenous insulin rapidly so that they are hypoglycaemic for a large part of the day. If, in these cases, the effect of an intermediate-acting insulin lasts only 12–18 h, a long-acting preparation can be tried. If the effect is less than 12 h, either a long-acting insulin can be used or the intermediate-acting insulin can be given at 12-hourly intervals.

The criteria used to diagnose these three causes of instability are shown in Table 17.8.

MANAGEMENT DURING SURGERY

If surgery is necessary (eg, for ovariohysterectomy) on the morning of surgery, no food is given and only half the daily insulin administered. During surgery, an intravenous infusion of 5% glucose is given and this is continued until the animal is eating again. Blood glucose is checked during and after surgery and, if necessary, soluble insulin can be given in small doses.

PROGNOSIS

With careful attention to detail a good quality of life can be maintained, in some cases for five or more years. Long-term complications are cachexia, persistent infections (especially cystitis), and in dogs diabetic cataracts. A less common complication is glomerulonephritis and rarely, diabetic retinopathy and diabetic neuropathy may occur.

Table 17.8 Serial blood glucose assays in the diagnosis of complex instability.

Insulin resistance	Blood glucose consistently >16 mmol/l throughout 24 h period
Insulin-induced hyperglycaemia	Rapid fall to <3.5 mmol/l following insulin injection followed by rise to >16 mmol/l
Rapid metabolism of insulin	Blood glucose >11 mmol/l within 18 h of insulin injection with minimum blood glucose of 4.5–5.5 mmol/l

REFERENCES

Chastain, C. B. & Nichols, C. E. (1984) *Veterinary Clinics of North America* **14**, 859.
Eigenmann, J. E. (1981) *Journal of the American Animal Hospital Association* **17**, 805.
Evans, J. M. & Sutton, D. J. (1988) *Journal of Small Animal Practice* **29**, 391.
Nelson, R. W. & Feldman, E. C. (1983) *Journal of the American Veterinary Medical Association* **182**, 1321.

CHAPTER 18

Clinical Use of Neuromuscular Blocking Agents in Dogs and Cats

GERARD BROUWER

INTRODUCTION

General anaesthesia is recognized as involving three principal effects: narcosis (unconsciousness), freedom from reflex response (analgesia) and muscle relaxation (Fig. 18.1). All three effects can be achieved using a single general anaesthetic drug such as thiopentone or halothane; however, effective muscle relaxation will only be obtained under deep levels of anaesthesia which tend to be accompanied by significant side-effects such as respiratory depression and circulatory failure.

Following the introduction of neuromuscular blocking agents in the 1940s, it became possible to produce the three effects of anaesthesia independently of each other by use of drugs which had virtually single actions in the body. A patient could now be maintained under light levels of anaesthesia with adequate analgesia and good muscle relaxation. Thus grew the concept of "balanced anaesthesia", its first use in veterinary practice being reported in 1954 by Hall and Weaver.

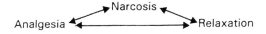

Fig. 18.1
Components of general anaesthesia.

ACHIEVING MUSCLE RELAXATION

During anaesthesia muscle tone can be abolished or reduced in a number of different ways.

Centrally acting drugs. General anaesthetics such as the barbiturates and the volatile agents, such as halothane and methoxyflurane, produce muscle relaxation by depression of the central nervous system leading to decreased activity of the ventral horn cells of the spinal cord. Profound muscle relaxation is achieved under states of deep central nervous system depression, but at the same time there is likely to be concurrent depression of the respiratory and vasomotor centres leading to respiratory and circulatory failure. Maintaining an unnecessarily deep level of anaesthesia cannot be recommended and may contribute to increased incidences of mortality and morbidity.

Local anaesthetics. When local anaesthetic agents are injected around nerves or into muscle masses, natural muscle tone is lost. While such muscle relaxation can be useful, the temperament of many animals prevents the use of local anaesthetics without combination with narcosis. Local anaesthetics are time consuming to administer, are not effective immediately and can have a protracted duration of action. In certain techniques the control of the circulatory system can be compromised through paralysis of sympathetic nerves. In the dog and cat their usefulness is limited, but should not be discounted especially as part of a balanced anaesthetic protocol in the sick or elderly patient.

Neuromuscular blocking drugs. These drugs, frequently referred to as "muscle relaxants" act at the neuromuscular junction producing relaxation or paralysis of voluntary striated muscle. They have no significant action in the body other than at the neuromuscular junction, and it is possible to produce rapid and reliable muscle relaxation without affecting the central nervous system or the circulation. It is the use of this group of drugs that will be considered now in greater detail. (While mephenesin and guaiacol glycerine ether are properly considered to be muscle relaxants, they exert their action at the synapses of the spinal cord; their clinical usefulness in the dog and cat is very limited, and will not be discussed further.)

INDICATIONS

Muscle relaxants are indicated for use in a variety of clinical situations:

(1)   To permit reduction to the amount of anaesthetic needed to achieve adequate operating conditions where muscle relaxation is not the main requirement, eg, in the sick or elderly patient

(2)   To relax skeletal muscles for easier surgical access, eg, laparotomy

(3)   To facilitate atraumatic endotracheal intubation in cats

(4)   To facilitate control of respiration during thoracic surgery

(5)   To provide improved conditions for bronchoscopy and endoscopy

(6)   To assist reduction of dislocated joints

(7)   To prevent reflex movement during delicate periods of surgery, eg, ophthalmic or aural procedures

In man, one of the principal indications for the use of relaxants is to facilitate controlled ventilation. It is recognized that it is important to avoid hypoxia and hypercarbia which tend to develop in the spontaneously breathing anaesthetized patient; thus it has become normal practice to control ventilation under anaesthesia with the aid of relaxants. The use of relaxants increases chest compliance and reduces resistance to ventilation so that lower ventilating pressures need to be applied. In veterinary clinical anaesthetic practice it is likely that animals too will develop hypoxia and hypercarbia insidiously when allowed to breath spontaneously under moderate levels of general anaesthesia, thus consideration might be given in the future to routine controlled ventilation with or without the use of muscle relaxants.

While it is helpful to use relaxants during the reduction of joint dislocations, clinical experience suggests that the reduction of fractures is seldom eased by their use.

CONTRAINDICATIONS

The use of muscle relaxants is specifically contraindicated in certain circumstances:

(1) When there is an absence of adequate facilities for administering intermittent positive pressure ventilation
(2) When there are doubts about the ability to assess the level of consciousness.

It needs to be emphasized that neuromuscular blocking drugs have no narcotic or analgesic properties. Therefore, it is *essential* to ensure beyond reasonable doubt that during any surgical procedure the animal is unconscious and incapable of appreciating pain or fear throughout the period in which the relaxant may be in use.

There are also some situations in which *caution* should be exercized in the use of relaxants:

(1) Where the animal is suffering from hypovolaemia
(2) Where there is evidence of electrolyte imbalance
(3) Where there is evidence of pre-existing liver or renal disease which could affect elimination and excretion of the drugs
(4) When the animal is suspected of suffering from myasthenia gravis

In these circumstances relaxants may still be used, but the dose schedules and selections of agents need particularly careful consideration.

NEUROMUSCULAR BLOCKING DRUGS

Two types of neuromuscular blocking drug can be used clinically in veterinary practice: depolarizing (non-competitive) and non-depolarizing (competitive) agents. A detailed discussion of the mechanism of neuromuscular blockade is beyond the scope of this article, but familiarity with the pharmacological actions of chosen relaxants is essential before an attempt is made to use them for the first time. Some of the range of available drugs are described below. NB. These are human drugs not licensed for animal use in the UK.

d-Tubocurarine chloride (Tubarine; Wellcome Foundation)

d-Tubocurarine is a non-depolarizing relaxant which is still used extensively in man, where it continues to be a safe and reliable agent. In veterinary anaesthesia it is far less useful. In the dog, d-tubocurarine causes a severe fall in blood pressure; this effect appears to be due to the release of histamine, and blocking of transmission of impulses across autonomic ganglia. The drug cannot be recommended for routine use in small animal practice.

Pancuronium bromide (Pavulon; Organon Teknika)

This is a widely used non-depolarizing agent which fulfils the need for a rapidly acting relaxant with few side-effects and a moderate duration of action. In both dogs and cats a dose of 0.06–0.1 mg/kg produces about 20–40 min relaxation according to the anaesthetic protocol. Pancuronium does not cause histamine release. Care should perhaps be taken in dogs suffering from chronic nephritis and other conditions that impair renal function because the drug, at least in part, is excreted unchanged in the urine. Pancuronium is a safe and reliable drug widely used in veterinary anaesthetic practice.

Gallamine triethiodide (Flaxedil; Rhône-Poulenc)

In dogs the injection of gallamine, a non-depolarizing relaxant like d-tubocurarine and pancuronium, does not appear to give rise to histamine release. However, there is a marked vagal blocking activity which causes a rise in heart rate by as much as 10–20% within 1.5 min of administration; the rise in heart rate may also be accompanied by a rise in blood pressure. It may have a weak inhibitory effect on liver cholinesterase enzyme production, and this action may be responsible for the transient decrease in blood pressure after intravenous injection in the cat but this appears to have little clinical significance.

In both dogs and cats doses of 1–2 mg/kg produce between 15–30 min relaxation. The agent is not detoxified in the body and is excreted unchanged in the urine; therefore, its use is contraindicated in animals with renal failure, and it should be used with caution in the presence of chronic nephritis. Occasional difficulties with reversal of the agent have contributed to its gradual disappearance from routine veterinary anaesthetic practice although it remains popular in some research laboratories.

Alcuronium chloride (Alloferin; Roche Products)

Alcuronium is a non-depolarizing drug free from significant histamine releasing or ganglionic blocking effects. Doses of around 0.1 mg/kg produce approximately 30–40 min relaxation in the dog and cat, characterized by an initial slow onset of action. Intravenous injection produces little change in heart rate, arterial pressure or central venous pressure. After repeated increments of alcuronium difficulties have been experienced with reversal of the blockade by neostigmine; therefore, it is suggested that the use of the drug is limited to those procedures that can be completed using just a single injection. Alcuronium is currently not in widespread use in veterinary practice.

Vecuronium bromide (Norcuron; Organon Teknika)

This is a non-depolarizing relaxant that is very similar to pancuronium. In dogs, a single dose of 0.05–0.1 mg/kg produces 20–30 min relaxation depending on the anaesthetic protocol. Postoperative nausea and vomiting, sometimes delayed for several hours, is occasionally noted and would seem to be an undesirable feature. Nevertheless, vecuronium is regularly used in several of the British veterinary schools and has proved to be a very practical drug, especially in the dog.

Atracurium besylate (Tracrium; Wellcome Foundation)

This is an increasingly popular non-depolarizing relaxant with few cardiovascular side-effects. The metabolism is unusual in that atracurium is metabolized in plasma by the Hofman elimination (reduction) process and to a lesser extent by ester hydrolysis. Thus the relaxant effects tend to wane spontaneously and the use of reversal agents, although generally to be recommended, seems not to be essential. Repeated doses of the compound have little cumulative effect, unlike most other relaxants. Atracurium seems particularly indicated where liver or renal function is impaired, and has been safely used in cases of myasthenia gravis. Reports of its use in cats are limited, but in the dog an initial dose of 0.3–0.5 mg/kg produces 20–30 min relaxation.

Suxamethonium chloride (Anectine; Wellcome Foundation)

This is the only relaxant of the depolarizing class in clinical use. The onset of action is characterized by a progressive wave of muscle fasciculations over the body; this being the effect of initial muscle stimulation caused by depolarization of neuromuscular end-plate which precedes blockade. Human patients complain of muscle pains after the use of suxamethonium; this is difficult to assess in animals, although obvious muscle damage causing stiffness or lameness is not observed. The muscle contractures are known to cause the release of potassium, and this may be associated with cardiac dysrhythmias. Therefore, the use of suxamethonium in animals with pre-existing hyperkalaemia or cardiac dysrhythmias may be unwise.

In the cat, a dose of 0.5–1.0 mg/kg lasts about 5 min. There is an immediate fall in blood pressure, followed by a rise to a point above the resting level. This fall in blood pressure is largely prevented by premedication with atropine. In the dog, doses of approximately 0.3 mg/kg achieve 10–20 min relaxation; there is usually a marked rise in blood pressure accompanied by bradycardia unless atropine premedication has been used, when a degree of tachycardia may occur through persistence of a nicotinic effect. Repeated doses of suxamethonium, especially when given before the effects of the previous dose have worn off, can lead to a potentiation of effects and a long period of blockade. Thus it might be preferable to select an alternative relaxant if the required period of relaxation is realistically going to exceed the duration of a single dose.

Suxamethonium is hydrolysed *in vivo* by plasma pseudocholinesterases. There is, therefore, no need to actively reverse depolarizing relaxants; indeed, the administration of anticholinesterases will enhance depolarization and potentiate the duration of action. Circulating levels of pseudocholinesterases are depressed by organophosphorus compounds (such as flea collars and some insecticidal sprays) and suxamethonium should be avoided if the animal is suspected to have been exposed to these agents in the recent past.

CLINICAL FEATURES IN THE USE OF NEUROMUSCULAR BLOCKING AGENTS

The sequence in which muscle groups become paralysed after administration of neuromuscular blocking drugs is relatively common in all animals.

Muscles of the face, jaw and tail
↓
Neck muscles and those of the distal limbs
↓
Proximal limb muscles
↓
Muscles of the pharynx and larynx
↓
Abdominal muscles
↓
Intercostal muscles
↓
Diaphragm

From this it might be supposed that it would be possible to titrate the level of neuromuscular blockade without necessarily affecting effective spontaneous ventilation. While it might be possible to achieve relaxation of the limbs without affecting ventilation, adequate relaxation of the abdominal muscles is also likely to result in some blockade of the respiratory muscles and, therefore, assisted ventilation would be required. In practice, it is very difficult to achieve such fine control of the level of relaxation, and it can be assumed that there always will be a need to provide intermittent positive pressure ventilation (IPPV).

Although dose rates have been given earlier for a number of the relaxant drugs, these are to be considered no more than guides. The response to a dose of relaxant depends on a variety of matters; the physique of the animal, its age and overall health, the normality of its neuromuscular transmission, acid-base balance, liver and renal function. Furthermore, it is well recognized that many anaesthetic drugs, including the volatile agents such as halothane and isoflurane, potentiate the effects of relaxants; the suggested durations of action given earlier could be extended by as much as 50–100% · depending upon the anaesthetic protocol adopted.

Certain antibiotics (eg, neomycin and streptomycin) are known to have slight neuromuscular blocking properties and may potentiate the action of relaxants. The use of these antibiotics is best avoided in the perioperative period.

Neuromuscular blocking drugs are normally given by the intravenous route and can initially be given in small increments until the desired degree of relaxation is achieved; the one exception being that the initial doses given to cats for endotracheal intubation need to be sufficient to abolish all laryngeal tone. During the procedure further doses of relaxant can be administered if muscle relaxation wanes; these supplementary doses should normally not exceed half the initial dose. Should additional muscle relaxation be required within about 30 min of the end of a procedure, it is probably better to achieve this by a slight increase in the depth of anaesthesia rather than give an incremental dose of relaxant.

The use of both depolarizing and non-depolarizing relaxants during the same procedure is *not* to be recommended. Care should be taken to select in advance the most appropriate relaxant for the proposed procedure according to its pharmacological actions and its duration of effect.

PRINCIPAL CONSIDERATIONS IN RELAXANT ANAESTHETIC TECHNIQUES

(1) The benefits arising from the use of muscle relaxants as part of a balanced anaesthetic technique can only be appreciated if relaxants are used in conjunction with light levels of central nervous depression, sufficient to ensure that the animal remains unaware throughout. This is achieved by careful combination of premedicants (which may include analgesics) and intravenous and inhalation anaesthetics; the choice is wide and can be influenced by personal preferences.

(2) There must be adequate provision for providing sustained IPPV. Manual ventilation is possible using a Modified Ayre's T-Piece, a Water's To-and-Fro system or a circle system; Magill, Lack or Bain systems are not really suitable for this purpose, although they can, of course, be used to ventilate the lungs in an emergency.

Mechanical ventilators are exceedingly useful. Many are adopted from human use; examples include the Manley ventilator and the Flomasta. The method of operation of mechanical ventilators varies considerably, and it is not possible to elaborate further here.

It needs to be emphasized that it is important to have a thorough understanding of how the anaesthetic systems and ventilators work before attempting to administer IPPV for real in an animal. How each system works determines fresh gas flow rates and gas compositions that should be used to administer IPPV and provide anaesthesia.

(3) A clear airway is required at all times and endotracheal intubation is to be considered *essential*. The absence of the pharyngeal and laryngeal reflexes, coupled with relaxation of the oesophageal muscles, make inhalation of regurgitated stomach contents all the more likely. Further, if IPPV is applied without intubation, the stomach and the intestines may become inflated.

(4) Given that muscle relaxants and reversing agents are given intravenously, the placement of an intravenous catheter at the start of the procedure should be considered mandatory to ensure an open vein at all times.

(5) Monitoring anaesthesia under neuromuscular blockage is a particularly skilled task which should not be delegated to anyone unless they are thoroughly familiar with monitoring

routine (spontaneously breathing) anaesthetics and have had additional training in relaxant anaesthetic techniques.

TECHNIQUE OF RELAXANT ANAESTHESIA

The precise technique adopted will depend on personal preference, the nature of the procedure, and the availability of drugs and equipment. Therefore it is only possible to provide a general outline in this paper.

PREMEDICATION

Premedication should always be considered as it allows reduction in the total amount of anaesthetic needed for induction and maintenance. A typical premedicant will be acepromazine, which may be combined with an analgesic such as pethidine or buprenorphine.

Premedication should also include an anticholinergic agent such as atropine to counter the side-effects of many of the relaxants which include marked salivation. Furthermore, atropine premedication will go some way towards offsetting the muscarinic side-effects (eg, increased salivation and bradycardia) of reversal agents such as neostigmine, even though additional doses are likely to be administered at the time of reversal.

At premedication or just prior to induction anaesthesia, a peripheral vein should be catheterized to ensure venous access throughout the procedure.

INDUCTION AND MAINTENANCE

Anaesthesia would normally be induced intravenously (eg, thiopentone or propofol) followed by endotracheal intubation; anaesthetic induction can then be completed with inhalational agents (eg, halothane or isoflurane in oxygen, and possibly supplemented with nitrous oxide). In certain cardiothoracic procedures it is advisable to commence IPPV soon after induction of anaesthesia and the relaxant is given at induction or as soon as intubation has been completed. More commonly the relaxant is given just prior to starting surgery to make best use of the period of paresis; IPPV is applied as soon as the relaxant takes effect.

The muscle relaxant is given by *slow* intravenous injection; the initial doses have been listed earlier, and these can be supplemented as the relaxant wanes with half dose increments as necessary.

IPPV is applied via an appropriate anaesthetic system (eg, T-Piece or To-and-Fro) or mechanical ventilator using oxygen alone (when anaesthesia is maintained intravenously) or using oxygen with nitrous oxide supplementation with additional low concentrations of volatile agent. Great care needs to be taken when ventilating with volatile anaesthetic agents since it is all too easy to overdose the animal; vaporiser settings should be *reduced* to a quarter or half the setting used if the animal was breathing spontaneously. Typical settings when ventilating with 30% oxygen and 70% nitrous oxide would be 0.2–0.5% halothane, 0.3–0.6% isoflurane or 0.1–0.2% methoxyflurane, but the precise settings would depend upon the needs of the animal. Attempting to ventilate with volatile agents without the use of a calibrated and regularly serviced vaporiser would be most unwise.

During IPPV it is important to ensure that ventilation is adequate for proper gas exchange. Each tidal volume should ensure good lung inflation, the chest wall moving slightly more than during spontaneous respiration. The ventilating rate should approximate to the normal respiratory frequency; 25–30 breaths/min in cats and 16–20 breaths/min in dogs. Indeed it is generally safer to slightly hyperventilate during relaxant anaesthesia than risk hypoventilation. Hyperventilation also potentiates the actions of nitrous oxide (if used), thereby allowing further reduction in the amount of supplemental anaesthetic required.

Some concern is expressed over the hypocapnia that hyperventilation might induce; limited periods of hypocapnia appear to have no clinical significance, but during prolonged procedures inspired carbon dioxide levels may be increased slightly by increasing the ventilatory deadspace or adding 3–4% carbon dioxide gas to the ventilating gas mixture.

Intubation of cats

The use of suxamethonium to facilitate endotracheal intubation
in the cat deserves special consideration. The relaxant is given
immediately following the intravenous induction agent. The
neck is extended, and while the relaxant takes effect the cat
is gently ventilated with 100% oxygen using a Modified
Ayre's T-Piece and a tight fitting facemask; only four to five
"breaths" are usually necessary. A large diameter lubricated
non-cuffed endotracheal tube can then be passed and tied
into place. The tube is then connected to the T-Piece and a
few further "breaths" of oxygen are applied. Gradually, the
oxygen can be replaced with a mixture of 30% oxygen and
70% nitrous oxide while ventilation is continued. Hyperventilation at this time will lower arterial carbon dioxide levels and
prolong apnoea unduly. Within five minutes, spontaneous
ventilation will resume and IPPV can be suspended; a normal
gaseous anaesthetic protocol can then continue. For the extra
effort involved, the technique provides excellent intubation
conditions.

MONITORING ANAESTHESIA

In the spontaneously breathing animal, the depth of anaesthesia can be monitored using a well established series of
techniques which might include some or all of the following:

(1) Testing jaw tone
(2) Assessing the pedal withdrawal reflex
(3) Noting of the position of the iris, the diameter of the
pupil and the strength of the palpebral reflex
(4) Assessing the respiratory rate, pattern and depth
(5) Noting the colour of the mucous membranes and assessing the capillary refill time
(6) Palpating the pulse; determining heart rate and assessing
pulse quality.

Under relaxants many of these indices cannot be used.
Under full blockade there can be no jaw tone, and the pedal
withdrawal reflex is inoperative if noxious or painful stimuli
are applied. The iris tends to remain central and paresis of

the muscles of the face means that there is no palpebral reflex; indeed, the appearance is that of a deeply anaesthetized animal. The pupil, however, remains constricted unless anaesthesia is excessively deep, but even this reassuring sign can be masked by the mydriatic action of atropine if it has been used for premedication. The lack of respiratory indices is perhaps most frustrating since respiratory rate and pattern are universally used, however subconsciously, by veterinary surgeons and nurses alike to monitor an anaesthetic.

Monitoring the colour of the mucous membranes now assumes greater importance. Inadequate ventilation can result in hypoxia and the development of a blue hue to the membranes; hypoventilation can also allow hypercarbia to develop, manifested by a characteristic cherry red coloration of the membranes. The mucous membranes also can be used to assess the circulation. Capillary refill time can continue to be used as an index of cardiac output; pallor can suggest hypovolaemia, shock, or vasovagal syncope in response to awareness of pain. Pulse rate and pulse quality continue to be essential parameters in assessing the level of anaesthesia.

Given the limitations, it is important to be extra diligent in monitoring anaesthesia under muscle relaxants, and particular attention should be given to signs of possible awareness.

Signs of awakening under muscle relaxants

(1) Increased pulse rate not related to haemorrhage or deliberate changes in the anaesthetic procedure
(2) Signs of vasovagal syncope; pallor of the mucous membranes, reduction in perceived pulse quality as a result of hypotension or peripheral vasoconstriction
(3) Increased metabolism as manifested by an increased end-tidal carbon dioxide level unprovoked by deliberate changes to the ventilating pattern or the composition of the inspired gases. (The use of capnographs, particularly in long procedures has much to be recommended)
(4) Lachrymation and increased salivation (even in the presence of anticholinergic premedication)
(5) The occurrence of slight muscle movements (of the face, tongue or distal limbs) in response to potentially painful

stimulation. Curling of the tip of the tongue is a characteristic sign.

Should anaesthesia be assessed to be too light, immediate steps should be taken to deepen anaesthesia by administering small increments of either inhalational or, preferably, intravenous anaesthetic. Should the problem persist then consideration should be given to administering an additional dose of analgesic.

NEUROMUSCULAR BLOCKADE

Given the variation in the response to a given dose of relaxant and rate of recovery from neuromuscular blockade, it would seem desirable to be able to monitor the nature and degree of blockade during anaesthesia. Unfortunately, many of the sophisticated systems used in the laboratory are quite impractical in the operating theatre environment. In recent years portable electromyographs and peripheral nerve stimulators have begun to be introduced into human operating theatres with some success; in veterinary anaesthetic practice such devices remain uncommon.

The peripheral nerve stimulator, with electrodes arranged to stimulate facial or distal limb muscles and delivering a "train-of-four" stimulation (Ali and others 1971) may be a useful device. The degree of blockade is assessed not necessarily by "twitch" strength but by the absence of one or more of the four grouped muscle contractions possible in each cycle. Nevertheless, such monitors only assess one muscle or group of muscles; the responses of other groups (including those of respiration) may well be different through differences in temperature and blood supply. Thus clinical judgement, based on the duration of apnoea under standard anaesthetic conditions, is equally as useful in the practical situation.

Signs of incomplete muscle relaxation

(1) Signs of spontaneous respiratory movements in spite of IPPV. Typical signs are slight diaphragmatic or abdominal efforts out of synchronization with the ventilator

(2)   Decreased chest wall compliance and increased resistance to ventilation. Manual ventilation will insidiously require slightly greater effort, while dials on some mechanical venti- lators will reveal that greater pressures are required to deliver the same tidal volume as before
(3)   Increased jaw muscle tone

It will be appreciated that less anaesthetic is required during anaesthesia combined with relaxants compared with conventional anaesthesia where the patient breathes spon- taneously, and sometimes one of the signs of waning neuromuscular blockade is a lightening of anaesthesia as well as the return of respiration.

Within 20–30 min of the end of the procedure, muscle relaxation is preferably increased by deepening anaesthesia a little. Otherwise, small increments of up to half the initial induction dose of relaxant may be given. During long periods of relaxation it is best to wait for signs of the relaxant wearing off before additional doses are given; giving timed doses irrespective of the actual degree of blockade risks generating a severe blockade which is subsequently difficult to reverse. Repeated doses of suxamethonium are best avoided.

REVERSAL OF MUSCLE RELAXANTS

Depolarizing muscle relaxants are not actively reversed; their effects are terminated naturally by the action of systemic pseudocholinesterase enzymes. Theoretically, non-depolariz- ing (competitive) muscle relaxants need not be reversed either since their effects would wear off in time; however, their duration of action is such that active reversal is usually a clinical necessity.

Three drugs used for the reversal of neuromuscular blockade include neostigmine, pyridostigmine and edrophonium. These act by inhibition of the enzyme acetylcholinesterase which is responsible for the normal destruction of acetylcholine. A convenient, if greatly simplified, explanation of the mode of action is that antiacetylcholinesterase compounds (simply termed "anticholinesterases") allow accumulation of acetylcho- line in the area of the post synaptic cholinergic receptor; in sufficient concentration, acetylcholine will compete for and replace the relaxant at the receptor and restore neuromuscular transmission. Of the three compounds, neostigmine methyl-sulphate (Prostigmin; Roche Products) appears to be the most widely used.

Anticholinesterases like neostigmine have additional actions at muscarinic receptors, leading to bradycardia, salivation, urination and defecation. These effects need to be counteracted by giving atropine intravenously in advance of the anticholinesterase; doses of 0.03–0.05 mg/kg atropine are normally used. In practice, provided that some atropine has been given during premedication, the additional amounts of atropine necessary can safely be mixed in the same syringe as the dose of neostigmine.

The action of the non-depolarizing muscle relaxant must start to wane before it can be safely antagonised with an anticholinesterase. For this reason it is recommended that reversal is not normally attempted within 20–30 min of the last dose of relaxant. Early reversal risks generating a blockade that becomes increasingly refractory to reversal attempts.

There is no universally agreed dose for neostigmine; many factors influence its effectiveness at reversing neuromuscular blockade, not least being the actual degree of blockade persisting at the time reversal is begun. Dose rates ranging from 0.01–0.1 mg/kg have been quoted. The recommended technique is to titrate the neostigmine to effect; in this way experience suggests that doses of 0.06 mg/kg neostigmine (combined with 0.03 mg/kg atropine) are commonly used.

Technique of reversal of neuromuscular blockade

Neostigmine (2.5 mg) and atropine (1.2 mg) are mixed together in the same syringe; using standard preparations, this provides about 3 cc of solution. Small aliquots of say 0.5 ml, are given by *slow* intravenous injection. After 1–2 min, ventilation is stopped for 10–15 s to see if spontaneous respiration will resume; if respiration is inadequate, IPPV is resumed and the test repeated 1–2 min later. Further aliquots can be given every 3–5 min. The dose of neostigmine should be supramaximal to ensure full reversal of all the effects of the relaxant, but generally doses of 0.1 mg/kg neostigmine should not be exceeded.

Great care should be taken to avoid hypoxia and hypercarbia while attempting to restore spontaneous respiration. Ventilation should be supported whenever there is any doubt about the effectiveness of respiration. The colour of the mucous membranes should be closely monitored for signs of hypoxia, and deliberate attempts to raise carbon dioxide tensions in order to stimulate respiration are to be thoroughly discouraged. The pulse should also be closely monitored; bradycardia should be treated with additional small doses of intravenous atropine if necessary.

A good time to reverse neuromuscular blockade is at the start of wound closure. Muscle relaxation is rarely required at this stage and the subsequent short period of spontaneously breathing anaesthesia allows time to assess that the effects of the relaxant have been properly reversed. The changeover from relaxant anaesthesia to spontaneously breathing anaesthesia should be as smooth as possible and may involve adjustments of the anaesthetic systems and anaesthetic gas mixtures. Thereafter, recovery from anaesthesia should be relatively routine by following conventional principles of monitoring and nursing care. Nevertheless the importance of ensuring that there is no residual blockade at the end of anaesthesia needs to be emphasized since weakness of the laryngeal and palatine muscles could result in respiratory obstruction once the endotracheal tube is removed.

Failure to restore spontaneous respiration

Persistent apnoea after attempted reversal of neuromuscular blockade can be caused by a number of factors:

(1) Overdose of relaxant. Excessive doses of relaxant or topping-up too frequently can lead to an unexpectedly severe blockade
(2) Misjudged reversal procedure. Attempts to reverse the effects of suxamethonium with an anticholinesterase, or administering neostigmine before the effects of a non-depolarizing relaxant have begun to wane, can cause a potentiation of the blockade rather than a reversal
(3) Central depression due to relative overdose with premedicant or anaesthetic drugs

(4)   Interference with excretion or elimination of relaxant. Liver and kidney disease can potentiate the duration of action of neuromuscular relaxants
(5)   Hypothermia. Changes in muscle and body temperature significantly affect the duration of action of muscle relaxants. IPPV techniques tend to predispose the patient to hypothermia unless positive measures are taken to prevent it, and hypothermia is possibly the commonest cause of prolonged apnoea after relaxant anaesthesia techniques
(6)   Electrolyte or acid-base imbalances

While apnoea persists, effective IPPV should be maintained and sufficient anaesthetic administered, if thought necessary, to ensure that the animal remains unaware in the event that there is residual blockade. The use of analeptics and respiratory stimulants should be avoided. Excessive doses of neostigmine should also be avoided; if suggested maximal doses have already been used, further doses of neostigmine are best avoided for 30–60 min while IPPV is continued. Intravenous fluid therapy should be instigated to encourage excretion of the relaxant, and the patient should be kept warm.

SUMMARY

Neuromuscular blocking agents have been used in clinical canine and feline anaesthetic practice for over 35 years. A wealth of experience has been gained in the use of relaxants, which have more than proved their worth particularly in the management of seriously ill and traumatized animals.

There remains a reluctance in general practice to adopt anaesthetic techniques involving relaxant drugs. This may be because of an absence of trained veterinary anaesthetists and the fact that veterinary surgeons, while operating on the animal, tend to entrust at least the maintenance of anaesthesia to a nurse or theatre assistant.

There is little doubt that relaxant anaesthetic techniques involve more effort, require a thorough knowledge of the pharmacology of the drugs to be used and call for a sound understanding of the mode of operation of the ventilating system selected. Nevertheless, the widespread availability of relaxants and relatively inexpensive ventilators might encourage veterinary surgeons to review their anaesthetic procedures. The goal should be the provision of the very best in anaesthetic practice, rather than settling for cheap and convenient alternatives which may not always serve the best interests of the animals.

REFERENCES AND FURTHER READING

Ali, H. H., Utting, J. E. & Gray, T. C. (1971) *British Journal of Anaesthesia* **43**, 473.
Hall, L. W. & Weaver, B. M. Q. (1954) *Veterinary Record* **66**, 289.
Hall, L. W. & Clarke, K. W. (1983) (eds) *Veterinary Anaesthesia*, 8th edn, London, Baillière Tindall.

CHAPTER 19

Behavioural Problems in Dogs and Cats

VALERIE O'FARRELL

INTRODUCTION

As many as one in five dogs have behavioural problems severe enough to cause their owners marked inconvenience, but only a small proportion of these owners consult their veterinary surgeon about the problem. This is probably because they doubt whether the veterinary surgeon is able to offer help. Also, they may fear the same ridicule or condemnation which they have received from friends or relatives; the strength of an owner's attachment to his or her dog is commonly belittled by others, who feel that the best solution to a problem dog is to dispose of it.

The view that "there are no bad dogs, only bad owners" is widespread and many owners of problem dogs feel guilty and ashamed. Sadly, the result is that the veterinary surgeon often first hears of the problem when the owner can no longer tolerate it. By then it may be too late, as the owner, having taken a painful decision to have the dog destroyed, may be unwilling now to embark on treatment which takes time and effort and whose results are not immediate. To avoid a crisis of this nature occurring, it is advisable to make regular inquiries about possible behavioural problems.

Judging by the relatively infrequent referral to specialists of cats with behavioural disorders, there is probably not the same need to inquire about unreported problems.

GENERAL CAUSES OF BEHAVIOURAL PROBLEMS

Behavioural problems are usually caused by a combination of factors (Table 19.1).

GENETIC

A general predisposition to behavioural problems may be inherited, mediated by such factors as a hyperreactivity of the autonomic nervous system. A tendency to specific problem behaviours, eg, chewing and fear of men waving things, also seems to be inherited.

HORMONAL

The influence of testicular hormones increases the likelihood of various problem behaviours in dogs and cats, for example aggression, roaming and urine marking.

Table 19.1 Factors causing behavioural problems.

Genetic
Hormonal
Elicitation of instinctive behaviour patterns
Stress
  Changes in environment
  Conflict
Learning
Owner attitudes

ELICITATION OF INSTINCTIVE BEHAVIOUR PATTERNS

Some normal behaviour patterns, eg, dominance aggression in the dog and urine-spraying in the cat, are often inconvenient to owners. In many instances, owners are unaware of the kind of stimuli which trigger such behaviour, especially if they themselves perceive the stimuli differently. For instance, an owner leaning over a dog to pat it probably sees this as a friendly gesture, whereas the dog could perceive it as a threat to its dominance and therefore as a provocation to attack.

STRESS

Stress can contribute to the development of behaviour problems by lowering the threshold for the elicitation of some normal behaviour patterns. For example, stress can make a dog more sensitive to dominance threats and therefore more likely to bite. Stress can also provoke inappropriate instinctive behaviour which serves to relieve tension ("displacement activities"), eg, tail-chasing, sexual mounting of inanimate objects or destructive behaviour in the owner's absence.

The most common causes of stress are changes in the environment and conflict. Dogs are more likely to be affected by loss of or separation from human or animal companions, while cats are more likely to be upset by alterations in their physical environment or addition of people or animals to the household or immediate neighbourhood.

Where conflict occurs and the animal experiences unpredictable, unpleasant events which it cannot avoid, stress-induced behaviour may appear. In a dog this may happen in a household where different family members, perhaps unwittingly, reward and punish the same behaviour or where one owner, perhaps because of his own personality problems, behaves inconsistently towards it.

LEARNING

Early experiences can permanently influence later behaviour. Puppies or kittens which are deprived of sufficient contact with their own species, perhaps through having been acquired by their new owners too early, may as adults show abnormal behaviour in relation to their own species; reproductive behaviour seems particularly sensitive to this kind of deficiency. In the same way, puppies and kittens lacking contact with human beings or with a normal domestic environment in the first four months of life may never make acceptable pets.

Although most owners are aware that the frequency of occurrence of some behaviour may be influenced by the pleasantness or unpleasantness of the events which immediately follow it and use this principle to alter their dogs' or, more rarely, their cats' behaviour, they are often not aware of the extent to which they inadvertently shape their pets' behaviour by the same means. Thus, a dog's barking on a car ride may be rewarded by the car getting nearer to an exciting destination, such as the start of a walk, revealing new and interesting sights and sounds as it goes along. In addition, dog owners often underestimate the reward value of their own attention; mildly scolding the dog may have the opposite effect to that intended.

OWNER ATTITUDES

It is important to take owners' attitudes into account, as they may have a crucial effect on prognosis and treatment. Often, owners behave towards their dogs or cats in a way which produces behavioural problems because they are using an erroneous model of how the animals' minds work. The owner's behaviour, however, is also often partly determined by his own personality and the nature of his emotional attachment to his pet. For example, an aspect of a dog's behaviour, eg, attacking visitors, may be highly inconvenient and the owner may seek help to alter it; at the same time, without even being aware of it, he may also be gratified by the dog's protective instincts and may reward and encourage the behaviour in subtle ways.

It is also common to see a high level of anxiety in an owner or disturbance within a family reflected in some form of hyperreactivity in the dog or cat. The anxiety is probably transmitted from human to dog by means of inconsistent communications from the owner, giving rise to a state of conflict in the animal.

TREATMENT

The role of non-veterinary specialists in the treatment of small animal behaviour problems is somewhat controversial. Some veterinary surgeons feel that they are best placed to treat these problems. While it is obviously essential that any contributory physical pathology be diagnosed and treated, it is arguable that in many cases a successful diagnosis and treatment of the behavioural component requires specialist knowledge of various branches of psychology, particularly learning theory, ethology and human clinical psychology. It follows that the client's interests are best served by close collaboration between psychologist and veterinary surgeon and by a system in which mutual consultation can easily take place.

At the moment many veterinary surgeons have to decide whether to try to treat a behavioural problem themselves or whether to refer the client to a specialist some distance away. A useful rule of thumb is that if the problem is serious, particularly if it is acute, with the client extremely distressed or euthanasia a serious possibility, it is better to refer a case. On the other hand, where the problem is less severe or longstanding and where the causative factors can be clearly identified, intervention by the veterinary surgeon can often prevent a more severe problem from developing.

The most effective treatment of a behaviour usually involves a combination of treatment methods.

SURGERY

Castration is the surgical technique most commonly employed. It may be appropriate where the problematic behaviour is related to male sexual behavour, eg, intermale aggression, urine marking and roaming. In cats, castration reduces the frequency of such behaviour in a high proportion (80–90%). However, in dogs the success rate is more variable (50–90%). Therefore, it is wise to test the probable effects of castration with an androgen antagonist such as delmadinone (Tardak; Syntex) before proceeding with surgery.

In both dogs and cats, castration should always be immediately followed by behavioural treatment, in order to ensure that the problem does not reappear.

MEDICAL TREATMENT

At the moment there are very few drugs licensed for the treatment of behavioural disorders in small animals. Megestrol (Ovarid; Pitman-Moore) is the most commonly used. Being a synthetic progestogen, megestrol is most effective in the elimination of behaviours related to male sexual drive. However, it also has central nervous system effects which influence mood and general tractability more markedly than does castration. Megestrol therefore should not be used as a pharmacological test of the probable effect of surgical castration. Furthermore, it may be effective in the treatment of some stress-related disorders, such as excitability or destructiveness in dogs or excessive grooming in cats.

There are drugs used in human psychiatry which have been found to be effective in the treatment of anxiety in small animals, most notably diazepam and amitriptyline. When using these drugs it should be borne in mind that: (a) they have not been approved for use with dogs or cats; (b) dogs and cats may show idiosyncratic and paradoxical reactions to them, so when the drug is first administered the animal should be kept under observation for 24 h; (c) the dosage may have to be carefully regulated to achieve anxiety reduction without undue sedation.

None of these drugs should be used as the sole method of treatment if neither the animal's environment nor the owner's behaviour towards the animal is altered; also, there is a reduced possibility of improvement in the first place and a higher risk of relapse when the drug is withdrawn. Such medication should be regarded as a short-term measure designed to assist psychological methods of treatment.

BEHAVIOURAL TREATMENT (Table 19.2)

A different treatment programme must be designed for each individual case. However, many successful programmes conform to the following broad outlines.

Table 19.2 Behavioural treatments.

Can triggering stimulus be eliminated	→ Yes →	Gradually reintroduce triggering stimulus while rewarding desirable behaviour
↓ No ↓		
Can undesirable response be prevented	→ Yes →	Encourage and reward alternative desirable response
↓ No ↓		
Ensure undesirable response is not rewarded	→ Then →	Reward alternative desirable response when it appears

Rewards

(1) Use as wide a range of rewards as possible
(2) Make rewards as desirable as possible
(3) Reward should accompany or immediately follow desirable behaviour with no delay
(4) Initially reward desirable behaviour every time, then gradually reward more intermittently

Punishments

(1) If possible, do not punish
(2) Never punish if problem is stress-related
(3) Use only punishments which seem unconnected with owner
(4) Punishment should accompany or immediately follow undesirable behaviour with no delay

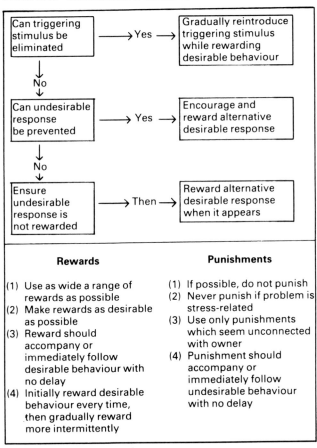

Elimination of undesirable behaviour

If the stimuli which trigger the undesirable behaviour have been identified, as far as possible the animal should not be exposed to them, so that, temporarily at least, the behaviour is not evoked. For example, a dog which is destructive in its owner's absence should not, for the time being, be left on its own.

If the provocative stimulus cannot be identified, or if it cannot be removed, the animal must be prevented from making the undesirable response.

Punishing a piece of behaviour is not a reliable way of eliminating it. If administered by the owner, punishment may actually make matters worse. It may increase the animal's general level of arousal, so making the animal more aggressive or anxious. In addition, a mild rebuke from an owner can often act as a reward. Punishment should therefore never be used when the undesirable behaviour is a reaction to stress or anxiety. If punishment is used, it is most effective if administered while the undesirable behaviour is going on, rather than afterwards, and if it appears to be unconnected with the owner, for example, a loud unpleasant noise or a water pistol.

Safer methods of eliminating a response are to prevent it just before it occurs, either physically or by distraction, or, if it does occur, make sure it is not rewarded.

Substitution of desirable behaviour

If it has been possible to eliminate the stimulus triggering the undesirable behaviour, it should be gradually reintroduced, the animal being rewarded for engaging in the desirable behaviour in its presence (Table 19.3). An important feature of this "systematic desensitization" is that the stimulus is reintroduced so gradually that the aggression, excitement or anxiety which gave rise to the problem behaviour is never evoked. If the problem behaviour is evoked, it is a sign that treatment is proceeding too quickly and should return to an earlier stage.

If it has not been possible to eliminate the triggering stimulus, then immediately after the undesirable response

Table 19.3 Guidelines to follow when using rewards to encourage good behaviour.

Rewards should be made as desirable as possible; for a dog, titbits can be effective, but must be really delicious, eg, cheese or chocolate, not biscuits.

As many kinds of rewarding experience as possible should be used. For a dog, not only praise and food can be rewarding but also, for example, having a ball thrown or being let out in the garden.

In order to be effective, rewards, like punishments, must accompany or immediately follow the behaviour they are intended to influence.

Initially the behaviour should be rewarded every time, until it is established. The rewards should then become gradually more intermittent.

has been stopped or prevented, the dog should be encouraged to engage in some alternative acceptable behaviour and rewarded for so doing. For example, a dog which had been distracted from chasing a cat might immediately be told to sit and given a titbit when it did so.

OWNER ATTITUDES

An owner's attitude to his pet is a personal matter and veterinary surgeons are often understandably wary of discussing these attitudes with their clients, even when these are clearly contributing to a behavioural problem. On the other hand, it is sometimes obvious that a problem will not be resolved unless the owner modifies his attitude. Sometimes an effective way of tackling this dilemma is to make a comment on a significant owner/dog interaction which is neither judgemental, eg, "you spoil that dog" nor vague, eg, "you should be firmer with him", but makes a factual observation about specific behaviour, eg, "it seems from what you tell me that you often reward the dog's barking by paying him attention" and makes a specific recommendation about how the owner should behave, eg, "try ignoring the dog when he pesters you for attention". This kind of comment has two advantages. It invites the owner to stand back and observe his own behaviour and thereby encourages him to review his whole attitude to the dog. It also offers specific

Table 19.4 Examples of specific behavioural disorders in cats and dogs, possible causes and treatment methods.

Disorder	Clinical picture	Possible causal factors	Possible treatment methods
Cats			
Urination in the house	It is important to distinguish *urine marking* from *normal urination*. Small quantities of urine sprayed on to a vertical surface are always urine marking, but occasionally it can take place in the squatting position. It is necessary to know the context in which urination occurs in order to make the distinction	*Urine marking* This is part of territorial behaviour and therefore is more common in entire than in castrated males and less common in females. It can be precipitated by a change of territory, eg, moving house, or by the addition of people or animals to the household *Normal urination* (or defecation) In the house this has no social connotations. In the absence of any physical disorder, it can be assumed that the cat has formed a preference for excreting in the house for one or more of the following reasons:	*Urine marking* (a) Castration of entire males (b) Megestrol acetate for females and castrated males (c) Reducing the territorial pressure, eg, by finding another home for one of the cats *Urination* (a) Possible causes should be eliminated (b) The cat may have to be retrained by keeping it under constant supervision and periodically escorting it outside or to a litter tray

(a) Going outside has become physically unattractive, difficult or frightening

(b) If the cat has a litter tray, the litter may be unappealing, either because it is unusual or it is not changed often enough

(c) If an inappropriate place is used once the smell may prompt the cat to use it again

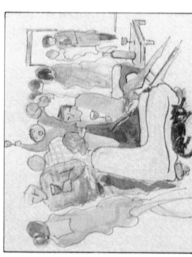

Fig. 19.1
Cats are more likely to be upset by the addition of people to the household.

Interspecies aggression

Territorial aggression can occur between adults of either sex. It can be distinguished from *intermale aggression* by the absence of preliminary threat rituals

Intermale aggression
(a) Castration
(b) If castration is ineffective or inappropriate, treat with megestrol

Territorial aggression
Treat behaviourally by initially keeping the cats apart and gradually exposing them to the sight, smell and sound of each other in rewarding circumstances

Table 19.4 Continued.

Disorder	Clinical picture	Possible causal factors	Possible treatment methods
Dogs			
Aggression towards people	Dog growls or bites when patted, groomed, displaced from its resting place, when an attempt is made to take something away from it or when someone enters its territory	(1) *Genetic* Disorder more common in certain breeds (2) *Hormonal* Particularly in male dogs and spayed bitches (3) *Instinctive* A dog which reacts aggressively is almost always trying to bring into line a perceived subordinate whom it sees as behaving in an inappropriately dominant way. The owner is often bewildered because he sees his own behaviour, eg, patting, as friendly rather than dominant	(1) *Hormonal* Megestrol acetate provides short-term relief and an opportunity for the owner to establish dominance (2) *Castration* This will reduce dominance within a few weeks in some cases. Where appropriate, it is valuable as a long-term measure, but its effect should be tested first pharmacologically (3) *Behavioural* (a) Avoid confrontations and situations where the dog is likely to feel threatened

(4) *Learning*
Unwittingly rewarding dominant behaviour, by letting the dog take the initiative and complying with its requests
(5) *Owner attitudes*
Owners may often have an anthropomorphic attitude to dogs and treat them as equals

(b) Establish dominance by ignoring the dog most of the time and paying attention to it only when it complies with a command
(4) *Owner attitudes*
Owners are often mystified as to how the aggression has arisen. They may be reassured when they realize their dog is neither mad nor bad, but is prompted by a normal instinct. They are often eager to try out a new regime. Occasionally, the aggression is part of a general psychological disturbance in the family, perhaps including physical abuse of the dog. The prognosis in these cases is much poorer

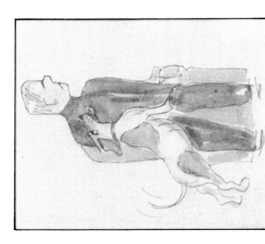

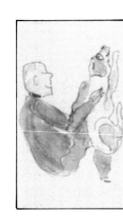

Fig. 19.2 The owner should establish dominance over the aggressive dog by ignoring it most of the time and rewarding it only when it complies with a command.

Table 19.4 Continued.

Disorder	Clinical picture	Possible causal factors	Possible treatment methods
Excitable behaviour	Dog appears excited or agitated; it may bark, dash to and fro or engage in idiosyncratic activity such as tail chasing. It may do this in specific situations, eg, in a car, or much of its waking life	(1) In severe cases, probably some constitutional abnormality, such as an inherited hyperreactivity of the nervous system (2) Usually, there is some precipitating stimulus. When the behaviour occurs occasionally, the stimulus may be obvious, eg, the door bell ringing. When the behaviour occurs more frequently it may be less easy to determine. One possibility which should be investigated is that the owner's presence is the precipitating factor (3) Such behaviour is usually maintained by some resultant reward; it may be that the behaviour is self	(1) *Isolate* the dog from the precipitating stimulus, then gradually re-expose it to the stimulus, rewarding it only for calm behaviour (systematic desensitization) (2) Where isolation from the stimulus is not possible, eg, if the stimulus is the owner, ensure excited response is never rewarded, eg, the owner should ignore the excitement. When it is not possible to ignore it, or when the response is self-rewarding, the dog should be *distracted* before it starts or, if necessary, physically prevented from continuing. When the undesirable

rewarding, eg, barking, or externally rewarded, eg, by attention from owner

(4) A high level of anxiety or conflict can make behaviour worse. Stress can be caused by inconsistent behaviour of the owner, who may oscillate between punishing the dog in exasperation and making a fuss of it to compensate

behaviour has stopped and the dog is calm, it should be rewarded

(3) Drugs

Tranquillizing drugs or megestrol may be useful in severe cases, especially where it is not possible to remove provoking stimulus

(4) Owner attitudes

Where behaviour is related to disturbance in the owner or family, it is often not helpful to point out this connection directly. Some owners, however, may be receptive to the idea that inconsistent behaviour on their part is stressful to the dog and may be able to modify their own behaviour accordingly

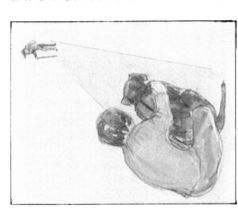

Fig. 19.3
Desensitizing a dog with a fear of men with sticks.

Table 19.4 Continued.

Disorder	Clinical picture	Possible causal factors	Possible treatment methods
Phobias	Dog trembles, cowers away or tries to escape from some stimulus, which is usually obvious, eg, thunderstorm or a veterinary surgeon, but in more severe cases this may be obscure, eg, dog is afraid to go outdoors	Often a genetic component. Early environment can also contribute. Prospective buyers of puppies should ask to meet the mother and ensure that the puppies have been reared in home surroundings. A traumatic incident or a series of less unpleasant incidents can in theory cause a phobia, but a convincing incident in the history is often hard to find	Initially, the dog should not be exposed to the frightening stimulus. Then a series of training sessions should be carried out in which the dog is made as calm as possible and is systematically densensitized to the feared stimulus by repeatedly presenting it in gradually increasing intensity. The aim of this treatment is never to provoke anxiety during the process
Destructive behaviour (a special case of excitable behaviour)	In the owner's absence, the dog chews furniture, loose objects, etc. It may also whine, urinate or defecate	Usually displacement activity caused by stress, resulting from separation from owners. Often, the dog is strongly attached to its owner and has not previously been accustomed to separation	(1) *Behavioural* Punishment is contraindicated as it is too late and it increases stress. Until the problem is treated the dog should not be left alone. It should be gradually desensitized to the owner's departure by first training it to assume a calm posture, eg, sitting in its basket, on command. This can be done by rewarding the response with praise, coupled with a food reward, which is gradually withdrawn as the behaviour

becomes established. When the dog will behave in a calm way on command, the owners should stage a series of mock departures gradually increasing in length; to begin with they should do no more than leave and then immediately return. If the dog is still calm on return, it should be rewarded; if not it should be ignored until it becomes calm. Once the dog can tolerate absences of half an hour it can normally be left safely for longer

(2) *Drugs*

Tranquillizing drugs or megestrol may be a useful adjunct to treatment, especially where owners have to leave their dogs while treatment is in progress

(3) *Owner attitudes*

Owners must be persuaded to abandon moralistic interpretations of the dog's behaviour, eg, "he knows he's done wrong; he looks guilty when I come back". The guilt in this case is fear associated with the owner's return and has no influence on the dog at the time of its destructive behaviour.

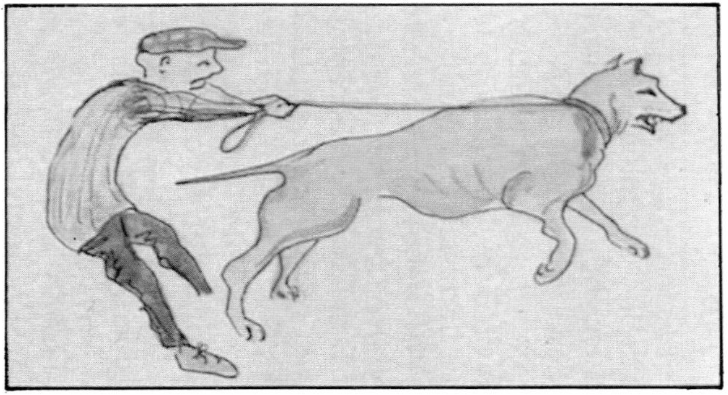

Fig. 19.4
Behavioural problems can be a source of great inconvenience and worry to the owner.

instructions which, when followed, often give rise to a change in attitude. For example, ignoring a dog for much of the time may itself reduce an owner's emotional involvement.

SPECIFIC DISORDERS IN DOGS AND CATS

Examples of specific behavioural disorders in dogs and cats, possible causes and treatment methods are listed in Table 19.4 (see also Figs 19.1–19.4). The main difference between the causes and treatment of behaviour disorders in these two species is that for cats social contact with their owners is less reliably rewarding. It is therefore less likely that any problem behaviour in a cat is the result of an owner inadvertently rewarding it and it is more difficult to teach it an alternative desirable response. On the whole, owner attitudes are of less significance with cats because the cat is less affected by them and because owners tend to have a more detached view of their cats.

FAILURE OF TREATMENT

Inevitably, treatment will fail in some cases. Often, this is because the owner is unwilling to spare the time and effort needed to produce change. Sometimes, the owner's personality prevents him from altering his own behaviour towards the animal. Sometimes, despite everyone's best efforts, it will prove impossible to modify the animal's behaviour. Occasionally, the behaviour is so antisocial, eg, an aggressive dog in a household with small children, that even a reduced likelihood of it occurring is unacceptable.

Even where success seems improbable, however, it is often worth trying to treat the disorder because (a) it is often hard to predict which cases will not respond to treatment—severity of the disorder is no guide; and (b) even when treatment fails and the animal has to be destroyed, an owner can often make this decision with greater peace of mind knowing that he has tried everything.

It should also be borne in mind that cure and euthanasia are not the only possible outcomes. Some owners can live more happily with a problem animal once they understand its behaviour. Also, where the problem is the result of mismatch between temperament of animal and owner, finding the animal a new owner can sometimes be a successful solution.

FURTHER READING

O'Farrell, V. (1986) *Manual of Canine Behaviour.* Cheltenham, BSAVA Publications.

Voith, V. L. & Borchelt, P. L. (1982) *Veterinary Clinics of North America* **12**, 4.

Voith, V. L. (1984) *Canine Medicine and Therapeutics* (ed. Chandler). Oxford, Blackwell.

Index

Abdominal injuries, 65 ff
Acanthosis nigracans, 262
Acepromazine, 6, 138 ff
Acetylcholine, 296
Adamantinoma, 230–1, 234–5
Adenocarcinoma, 199, 201
Adenoma
  hepatoid gland, 199
  sebaceous, 199
Adrenaline tartarate, 5–6
Adrenocorticotrophic hormone, 252
Aggression in cats, 311
Aggression in dogs, 312–3
Alcuronium chloride, 286
Alfentanyl, 144
Alloferin, 286
Alopecia
  growth hormone responsive, 254
  hormonal, 245 ff
  hormonal: feline, 259–60
  progesterone induced, 256
Alphaxalone/alphadolone, 144
Ameloblastoma, 230, 232, 234–5
Amitriptyline, 306
Ampicillin, 36, 63
Anaemia, 248
  non-regenerative, 178
Anectine, 287–8
Articular fractures, 59, 93
Association for the Study of
  Osteosynthesis, 100
Atracurium besylate, 287
Atropine, 20, 141, 143, 287, 291, 294,
  297
Atropine sulphate, 5–6
Avulsion fractures, 59, 92

Basset hound, 200
Behavioural problems, 301 ff
  effect of early experiences, 303
  excitable behaviour, 314 ff
  instinctive, 304
  owners causing, 304–5, 309, 313, 315,
    318
  phobias, 316
  punishment, 307–8
  reward treatment, 307, 309
  stress causing, 303
Bemegride, 5–6
Betamethasone, 49–50
Biliary tract trauma, 68 ff
Bladder, 67–8
Blindness, 19
Blood sampling, 169
Bone marrow
  aspiration and biopsy, 177 ff
  core biopsy, 185 ff
Boston terrier, 200
Boxer, 200, 210–11
Brain damage, 14 ff
Brietal, 144
Bull mastiff, 200
Buprenorphine, 6, 31, 139 ff, 144
Burns, 21
Butorphanol, 139, 144

Calcium borogluconate, 4 ff
Calcium chloride, 4, 6
Carcinoma
  basal cell, 199, 206, 230 ff
  squamous cell, 199, 206–7, 219, 223,
    225–7, 229, 235 ff

Cardiac arrest, 4
Cardiac tamponade, 42
Casts, 118 ff
    removal, 125–6
Cataracts, 267, 278
Catheterization, 2–3, 5, 11
Cellamin, 120 ff
Cephalic blood sampling, 170 ff
Cerclage wire, 98 ff
Chemotherapy
    in treatment of skin tumours, 206
Chlorpromazine, 11
Chow, 254
Cimetadine, 214
Clonezapam, 16
Cocker spaniel, 200
Corticosteroids, 249
Cranial decompression, 50
Cryosurgery, 226 ff
Cryptorchidism, 255
Cushing's disease, 250, *and see*
    Hyperadrenocorticism
Cyclophosphamide, 214

d-Tubocurarine chloride, 285
Dachshund, 210, 267
Delmadinone, 306
Delta Cast, 120 ff
Dermisol, 77
Devosteon, 273
Dexadreson, 5
Dexamethasone, 5 ff, 49–50
Dexon, 33
Diabetes mellitus, 260, 262 ff
    diet, 274–5
    owner education, 271, 276
Diaphragmatic rupture, 31 ff
Diaphyseal fractures, 92
Diazepam, 4, 16, 138 ff, 144, 306
Digoxin, 6
Diprenorphine, 140
Domitor, 144
Dopram-V, 5
Doxapram hydrochloride, 5–6
Dwarfism
    pituitary, 253
Dynamic compression plate, 106–7

Edrophonium, 296
Ehemer sling, 55–6

Emphysema
    subcutaneous, 40, 42
Epiphyseal separations, 63, 95
Epithelioma
    sebaceous, 199
Epulide, 223, 227, 229 ff
    acanthomatous, *see* Carcinoma, basal
        cell
Etorphine, 139–40, 144
External skeleton fixation, 113 ff

Fanconi syndrome, 268
Fentanyl, 139, 144
Fibroma, 199, 230 ff
Fibrosarcoma, 199, 208–9, 219, 223, 227,
    229, 238–9
Finger splints, 114–5
Flail chest, 29–30
Flamazine, 87
Flaxedil, 285–6
Fluanisone, 140, 144
Foam troughs, 132–3
Foam wedges, 132 ff
Fortral, 144
Fracture fixation, 58 ff, 91 ff
    articular, 59, 93
    avian, 128 ff
    avulsion, 59, 92
    diaphyseal, 92
    growth plate, 93
    healing time, 111
    jaw, 48
    neurocranial, 49
    reduction, 116
    rib, 31
    shaft, 59 ff, 98
Frostbite, 21
Furosemide, 6

Gallamine triethiodide, 6, 285–6
German shepherd, 253
Glomerulonephritis, 278
Glucagon, 264
Glucophage, 273
Glucorticoid, 266
Glycosuria, 265
    stress, 266, 268
Greyhound toe injuries, 53
Growth plate fractures, 93
Guaiacol glycerine, 282

Guar gum, 275
Gutter splints, 115–6
Gynaecomastia, 254, 256
Gypsona, 120 ff

Haemangioma, 199
Haemangiopericytoma, 199, 219
Haemangiosarcoma, 199
Haemoperitoneum, 66
Haemothorax, 43
Halothane, 281–82, 290 ff
Hartmann's solution, 2, 11, 271
Heart: ultrasound, 151, 163 ff
Heparin, 6
Hexcelite, 120 ff
Histiocytoma, 210
Horner's syndrome, 16
Hyperadrenocorticism, 250 ff, 257, 266, 268
Hypercalcaemia, 178, 201
Hyperoestrogenism, 258–9
Hyperpigmentation; 247–8, 250, 253 ff
Hyperplasia, 250
Hyperthermia
    in treatment of oral tumours, 223, 226 ff
    in treatment of skin tumours, 205 ff
Hyphema, 19
Hypnorm, 140, 144
Hypnovel, 144
Hypoglycaemia, 269, 275–6
Hypothyroidism, 247, 250, 253, 257

Immobilon
    Small Animal, 140, 144
Injury
    assessment, 1 ff, 8 ff
    management, 1 ff, 9 ff
Insulin, 264, 266, 271 ff
    resistance, 277–8
Interfragmental compression, 101–102
Intestinal tract injuries, 70
Intramedullary fixation, 96 ff
Intrapentone, 144
Ionising Radiation Regulations 1985, 131, 136
Iridodialysis, 19
Isoflurane, 291–92
Isoprotenarol hydrochloride, 6

Jaw fractures, 48
Jugular blood sampling, 170, 172 ff

Keeshond, 254
Ketamine, 141 ff
Ketonuria, 265
Kidney
    ultrasound, 152, 157–8

Laminectomy, 51
Leg injuries, 54
Leucocytosis, 178
Lignocaine hydrochloride, 5–6
Lipoma, 199
Liposarcoma, 199
Liver
    ultrasound, 151, 154 ff
Lymphoma, 206, 214, 215
    histiocytic, 218–9
Lymphoproliferative disease, 178
Lymphosarcoma, 178
Lysodren, 252

Male feminizing syndrome, 255–6
Mannitol, 6, 16, 49
Mast cell tumour, 199, 206 ff, 219, 242
Mechlorethamine, 217
Medetomidine, 138, 144
Medroxyprogesterone acetate, 265
Megestrol, 306, 310 ff, 317
Megimide, 5
Megoestrol acetate, 266
Melanoma, 199, 209–10, 219, 223, 226, 229, 240–1
Melolin, 86
Mephenesin, 282
Metformin, 273
Methadone, 139 ff
Methohexitone, 142 ff
Methotrimeprazine, 140
Methoxyflurane, 282
Methylprednisolone sodium succinate, 5–6
Metronidazole, 45
Midazolam, 138, 140–1, 143–4
Mitotane, 252
Modified Ayre's T-Pieces, 290, 292–3
Morphine, 139, 144
Morphine hydrochloride, 6
Morphine sulphate, 31

Muscle relaxation, 282 ff
  reversal, 296 ff
Mustargen, 217
Myasthenia gravis, 284, 287
Mycosis fungoides, 215 ff, 219
Myelodysplasia, 178
Myeloma, 178
Myeloproliferative disease, 178
Myocardial contusion, 43

Naloxone hydrochloride, 5–6
Narcan, 5
Neomycin/polymixin/bacitracin, 87
Neoplasia
  lymphoid, 178
Neoplasms
  cutaneous, 197 ff
Neostigmine, 286, 291, 296 ff
Neostigmine methylsulphate, 297
Nephritis, 285–6
Neurocranial fractures, 49
Neuromuscular blocking agents, 281 ff
  reversal, 298
Neuropleptanalgesia, 142
Neutralization plate, 107–8
Neutropenia, 178
Nikethamide, 5–6
Nitrous oxide, 292–3
Norcuron, 286

Obesity, 266–7, 273
Ocular trauma, 19 ff
Oesophagus, 44–5
Oestradiol, 259
Omnopon, 144
Orthopaedic injuries, 47 ff
Osteosarcoma, 239
Ovarid, 306
Owners causing behavioural problems,
  304–5, 309, 313, 315, 318
Owners of injured animals, 9–10

Pancuronium bromide, 285–6
Pancytopenia, 178
Papaveretum, 139 ff, 144
Papilloma, 199
Pavulon, 285
Penicillin, 77
Pentazocine, 6–7, 11, 31, 139 ff, 144

Penthidine hydrochloride, 6, 11, 31,
  139 ff
Peritoneal lavage, 70 ff
Pethidine, 139 ff, 144
Phenergan, 6
Pilomatricoma, 199
Pituitary dwarfism, 253
Pituitary tumour, 250, 253, 266
Plasmacytoma, 242
Plastrona, 120–1
Plate fixation, 102 ff
Pleural effusion, 189, 194–5
Pneumothorax, 37 ff, 52, 189
Polycythaemia, 178
Polyglactin 910, 33
Polyglycolic acid, 33
Pomeranian, 254
Poodle, 240, 267
  miniature, 254
Potassium chloride, 5–6, 21
Potassium gluconate, 21
Prednisolone, 214
Procaine hydrochloride, 5
Progesterone-induced alopecia, 256
Progestogen, 266
Proligestone, 273
Propofol, 142 ff, 291
Prostate
  ultrasound, 159 ff
Prostigmin, 297
Pug, 241
Pulmonary contusion, 35 f
Pyothorax, 190
Pyridostigmine, 296

Radiation
  in treatment of oral tumours, 226 ff
  in treatment of skin tumours, 204 ff
Radiography
  thoracic, 24
  dorsoventral thorax positioning,
    135–6
  lateral thorax positioning, 133
  restraint
    chemical, 136 ff
    physical, 131 ff
  ventrodorsal pelvis positioning, 134–5
Rapifen, 144
Rapinovet, 144
Respiratory distress, 23

Retriever, 238
  flat-coated, 201
  labrador, 200
Revivon, 140
Rib fracture, 31
Ringer's solution, 2, 11, 271–72
Road accidents, 1 ff
Robert Jones bandage, 55, 93–4, 113–4, 127
Rompun, 144
Rottweilers, 267

Saffan, 142 ff
Sam Splint, 115
Samoyeds, 267
Sandbags, 132 ff
Saphenous vein for blood sampling, 175
Sarcoma
  anaplastic, 226
  poorly differentiated, 239–40
  soft tissue, 208–9
  spindle cell, 239–40
Savlon, 4
Scalds, 21
Schnauzer, 200
Scotchcast Plus, 120 ff
Scotchflex, 120 ff
Scottish terrier, 200
Seborrhoeic dermatitis, 247, 250
Self mutilation, 87
Sertoli cell tumour, 254–5
Shaft fractures, 59 ff, 98
Shock, 12 ff
Silver sulphadiazine cream, 87
Skin grafting, 75 ff
Skin tumours, 197 ff
  biopsy, 203
Sodium bicarbonate, 4 ff
Sodium penicillin
  crystalline, 6
Soffban, 117
Solu-Medrone V, 5
Spinal cord damage, 14 ff
Spinal injury, 50 ff
Spleen, 66–7
  ultrasound, 159
Streptomycin, 77
Stress, 303, 306
Sublimaze, 144

Suxamethonium chloride, 287–8, 293, 296, 298
Synachthen, 252

Tachycardia, 13
Tardex, 306
Temgesic, 144
Tension band wiring, 101
Terriers, 267
Thiopentone, 142 ff, 281, 291
Thomas extension splint, 56–7, 93–4, 126–7
Thoracic injuries, 23 ff
Thoracocentesis, 24 ff, 40, 43, 189 ff
Thorax
  ultrasound, 167
Thrombocytopenia, 178, 187
Thrombocytosis, 178
Thyrotrophic hormone, 249
Thyroxine, 249
Torbugesic, 144
Torbutrol, 144
Torgyl, 45
Tracrium, 287
Travase ointment, 77
Trichoepithelioma, 199
Tubarine, 285
Tumour
  mast cell, 199, 206 ff, 219, 242
  melanocytic, 209–10
  oral, 223 ff
  pituitary, 250, 253, 266
  Sertoli cell, 254–5
  skin, 197 ff

Ultrasound, 147 ff
  heart, 151, 163 ff
  image interpretation, 153
  kidney, 152, 157–8
  linear array, 150
  liver, 151, 154 ff
  prostate, 159 ff
  spleen, 159
  thorax, 167
  transducer, 148 ff
  transducer: sector, 150–1
  uterus, 161 ff
Undercast padding, 117
Urination
  inappropriate

in cats, 310–1
Urine marking
   in cats, 310
Uterus
   ultrasound, 161 ff
Uveitis, 10

Valium, 144
Vecuronium bromide, 286
Velband, 86, 123
Velpean sling bandage, 57–8
Vetalar, 144
Vetcast, 94

Vetrap, 86
Vicryl, 33

Water's To-and-Fro System, 290, 292
Weimaraner, 200
Wounds, 20–1, 31
   penetrating, 27 ff, 39

Xylazine, 138–9, 143–4
Xylazine/ketamine combination, 143

Zimflex, 94
Zimmer splints, 114–5